LIFE-SAVING

HEALTH

SECRETS

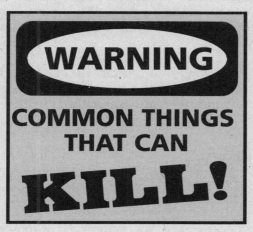

WARNING

COMMON THINGS THAT CAN

KILL!

JJ DeSpain

Publications International, Ltd.

JJ DeSpain writes about health, consumerism, and senior issues for national magazines in the United States and Canada. She is a former critical care nurse and spent three years as a respiratory therapy director in several nursing homes.

Louis Weber, CEO
Publications International, Ltd.
7373 North Cicero Avenue
Lincolnwood, Illinois 60712

Permission is never granted for commercial purposes.

Manufactured in U.S.A.

8 7 6 5 4 3 2 1

ISBN: 0-7853-4686-4

Contents

Introduction

Today, it seems that everything can hurt us. The air we breathe, the sun that warms us, the food we eat, and the medications we take all have the potential to cause serious harm. But those are just some of the dangers we encounter on a daily basis. Here are some sobering statistics:

- There are 76 million food-borne illnesses each year, causing 325,000 hospitalizations and 5,200 deaths.

- New treatments and medications can reduce or reverse the effects of stroke if they are administered within 90 minutes. But 58 percent of all stroke victims wait at least 24 hours to seek help.

- An average load of wash can leave 100 million *E. coli* bacteria in the washing machine.

- Every year, 56,000 auto accidents are caused by sleepy drivers; 40,000 people are injured, and 1,500 die as a result.

- More than 6,000 people die from a chemical- or medication-related poisoning each year, and 300,000 sustain disabling illnesses. And it's not just kids. The second highest risk category is adults aged 25 to 44.

- Nearly 50,000 cases of malignant melanoma are diagnosed each year, and 20 percent of those diagnosed will die from the disease.

- About 400,000 people are treated in emergency rooms every year from injuries from lawn and garden equipment.

- Drug errors are responsible for 7,000 deaths annually.

Some dangers, of course, are out of your hands. You simply can't control whether the driver next to you falls asleep at the wheel or whether your waiter washed his hands before he served your food.

But you can avoid many of life's hazards. It just takes knowledge and know-how, both of which you'll find in the following pages. The information and advice in *Life-Saving Health Secrets* will make you savvy about everything from eating out and cooking at home to traveling safely. You'll discover how to avoid fatal medical errors and how to keep your house safe from intruders. No matter where you are or what you're doing, *Life-Saving Health Secrets* can tell you how to protect yourself.

There's an old saying that a little knowledge is a dangerous thing. Well, this book offers a lot of knowledge, and that's the best security you can buy.

What's Cooking?

Lions and tigers and bears... well, not exactly. But the bacteria living in your kitchen can be just as dangerous—maybe more so since they can't be seen, smelled, or tasted. It's estimated that those little critters are responsible for 76 million food-borne illnesses each year, as well as 325,000 hospitalizations and 5,200 deaths. Food poisoning can be more than an inconvenient bellyache. In some cases it's a killer, originating, most often, right in our own kitchen. The good news is that food poisoning is preventable.

Guess What's Coming to Dinner

Up to 250 different kinds of uninvited guests, if you're not careful. Food poisoning symptoms can start as soon as 30 minutes after eating or not until several weeks after eating the tainted food. Often-times, food poisoning is confused with a viral infection or the flu. The following will help you determine whether you have food poisoning and what the source might be:

BACTERIAL FOOD POISONING
(This type of food poisoning is the result of spoiled or undercooked food.)

- diarrhea or frequent stools, often bloody and/or explosive

- fever

- severe abdominal cramps

- vomiting

BOTULISM

(This type of food poisoning is the result of foods that are incorrectly preserved or canned.)

- nausea, vomiting, diarrhea

- blurred vision, drooping eyelids

- dry mouth, difficulty swallowing

- difficulty breathing

- muscle weakness or paralysis

CHEMICAL TOXINS

(These are found in certain foods such as mushrooms, moldy peanuts, and potato sprouts.)

- vomiting, diarrhea

- dizziness

- mental confusion

- sweating

- watering eyes

- stomach pain

Five Food Poisoning Symptoms You Shouldn't Ignore

Botulism will kill you if you don't kill it first. So will some forms of chemical poisoning. Call 9-1-1 or get

Buffet Beware!

When serving a buffet meal at home, keep hot foods over a heat source and cold foods on ice. Never eat from a buffet or salad bar if the foods aren't maintained at the proper temperature; room temperature is never proper for anything perishable.

to the hospital immediately if you're experiencing the following symptoms:

- muscle weakness
- swallowing and breathing difficulties
- mental confusion
- blurred vision
- severe abdominal pains

You don't have time to sit around and hope the symptoms will go away.

FOOD-POISONING DIET

Milder cases of food poisoning won't kill you, but the symptoms can be unpleasant just the same. If you understand that the vomiting and diarrhea are your body's way of washing the bacteria out of your system, you might be able to tolerate it better. Dehydration should be your biggest concern. For mild symptoms, don't eat solid foods. First, try sipping clear liquids (water and sports drinks are the best choices because they keep essential body chemicals in balance). Continue drinking them for 12 hours after they stay down. Next, try eating rice, cooked cereals, crackers, and broths. Stick with the diet for 24 hours before you return to your normal eating habits.

WHO SHOULD BE EXTRA CAREFUL?

If you eat food, you're at risk for coming down with a food-borne illness. But some people are more at risk than others because their immune systems aren't functioning optimally, making them unable to fight off illness-causing bacteria. Particularly at risk are young children whose bodies are still developing immunity to diseases, older people whose immunity has decreased with age, pregnant women whose immune systems are working for two and are over-taxed by the extra work, and people with immune deficiency diseases, such as HIV/AIDS or cancer, who simply don't have enough immunity left in their bodies to fight.

Pesticides and Parsnips

In Doubt?

If in doubt, throw it out; if in doubt in a restaurant, send it back. When it's not cooked completely and its juices have flowed onto your veggies, ask for new veggies.

If it's been growing in the field, it's probably been sprayed with a pesticide that prevents, destroys, or repels insects, rodents, weeds, mold, and bacteria. This means that if you sneak a strawberry out of the bin in the produce department and eat it without first washing it, you've consumed some pesticides.

Luckily, the government controls the types and amounts of pesticides used on food crops, and the level of pesticide residue we consume in our foods normally is not harmful.

Still, you probably don't want to consume too many pesticides if you can help it. The best way to keep them out of your diet is simply to wash and scrub fruits and vegetables under running

Watch Those Sprouts

Raw sprouts can be harmful to your health—even deadly. The warm, humid conditions required for growing bean sprouts are also a rich breeding ground for bacteria such as *Salmonella* or *E. coli*. Only high temperatures will prevent bacterial growth, but they also keep the seeds from sprouting. So, for safety's sake, avoid raw sprouts; tossing them in your stir fry, however, should kill the troublesome microorganisms.

water. That will remove bacteria and traces of chemicals. Don't use household soap, as it's not meant for human consumption and can also cause an upset stomach. Peeling, throwing away the outer leaves, and trimming also gets rid of surface residues.

Those new produce washes on the market will do the trick, too, but according to recent government studies, they're not any better than plain old water and a good, hard scrub. And they have to be washed off as well, since they are primarily made of bitter tasting citric acid and baking soda. If you're sticking to the dietary guidelines and eating at least five servings of fruits and vegetables a day, produce washes require a lot of extra effort and expense, but they're growing in popularity anyway.

You can also choose to buy organic produce, which is grown and processed without synthetic pesticides. The cost is about 20 percent higher, but the upside is that you know what you are, or aren't, getting when you prepare those parsnips.

For more information, visit the EPA Web site at www.epa.gov/pesticides/food or write to the U.S. Environmental Protection Agency, Office of Pesticide Programs, 401 M Street, SW, Washington, DC 20460.

Lead Them Not Into Temptation

Lead from your coffee mug could kill you. Or, it could cause intestinal problems, anemia, and hearing loss. If you're using an imported mug or dinnerware that's marked "Not for food use" or "Decorative purposes only," stop doing so immediately! It's full of lead. Be particularly leery of any pottery-based product from Mexico, whether it's marked or not. Mexican pottery is notorious for lead contamination. So pour out the coffee and use that mug to hold pencils.

To avoid the risk of lead poisoning:

- Don't prepare, store, or serve foods in containers that may contain lead.

- Be wary of those prized antique mugs. Generally, lead wasn't used in commercial ceramic production after 1900, but many hobbyists and independent ceramic producers didn't get the message.

- Avoid leaded crystal as a storage container. It's wonderful as a serving dish, and you certainly want to drink your champagne from those beautiful lead-crystal flutes, but there is a small risk of lead contamination when food or beverages come in contact with it over an extended period of time. So, serve from the crystal, then use a storage container for leftovers.

To Market, to Market

If the juices from your raw meat trickle onto your apples, your apples could be contaminated with *Salmonella, E. coli,* and other microorganisms that can infect other food items. One bite of that crispy apple could make you sick from a meat contaminant.

Food safety begins well before you get home from

Groceries at Risk!

Don't put perishable groceries in a hot trunk. By the time you get home, the bacteria will already be producing their own stage show, and your intestinal tract is the intended stage. Keep them inside the car, and if your drive home takes more than 30 minutes, pack them in a cooler.

the grocery store. If you shop carefully, you can avoid unwittingly bringing home disease-causing bacteria. Microbes are lurking everywhere, including your grocery cart, especially if you don't take appropriate precautions. The following are some simple ways to cut

Microwave Safety

If you don't clean out the remains of things that pop and splatter in the microwave oven, they'll serve as a picnic ground for bacteria. You probably already know that, but you may not know that containers not labeled "microwave safe" may release chemicals into food when heated. So skip the butter tubs and anything else not specifically meant for the microwave, including the foam packing trays that meat comes on.

Plastic wraps, with the exception of those designated for the microwave, come with the same caution, so don't let them touch the food when you microwave.

You may also not know that when water is heated to the boiling point in the microwave, it sometimes appears calm, as if it's not really boiling. But it is boiling, and it can blow up and out of the container, causing serious burns if you jiggle the container. This happens because energy built up in the superheated liquid doesn't release normally through vapor, steam, or bubbles. Energy needs a point of escape, and for some reason it doesn't always get it in microwave heating. Moving the container or the contents creates a steam bubble, releasing the energy, which can cause the liquid to shoot straight up. To avoid this, stick something in the mug to diffuse the energy and create that opening, such as a tea bag or wooden stick.

down on contamination before you leave the store:

- Keep the juices from raw meats off all your other groceries. Grab some plastic bags to separate your meats and poultry from other foods as you shop.

- Reduce microorganisms by giving them the big chill. Buy cold and perishable foods last and get them to your refrigerator within an hour to prevent those nasty bugs from thawing out. If you can't get your food home within an hour, stick it in a cooler.

- Don't buy frozen foods unless they are frozen solid. And select frozen products, including meats, from the bottom of the case and refrigerated items from the back of the case, where it is coldest.

- Don't buy those pre-stuffed whole birds. Stuffing is a breeding ground for microorganisms that may not all cook out.

- Avoid canned foods with bulges or cracks. These could be signs of food poisoning inside— namely, botulism.

Store That Stuff the Right Way

In just two hours, 100 bacteria can divide into 24,600. That's why it's essential for your refrigerator and freezer to be working properly. You may think they're set to the right temperature, but have you checked lately? If you've accidentally bumped the thermostat in your refrigerator or freezer, temperatures can change. Take a look occasionally, especially if you think the food inside is spoiling too quickly or seems too warm to the touch. The danger zone in which microorganisms breed falls between 40°F and 145°F.

Some other storage suggestions:

- Don't store eggs and milk in the built-in door racks. These areas are the warmest in the fridge.

- Store fresh meat in the bottom of the refrigerator, and keep it in a plastic bag or on a plate to prevent the juices from dripping onto the shelf.

- Extreme temperatures and moisture can be harmful to canned goods and can promote bacterial growth, so store them in a cool, dry area.

For more information, visit the Web site of the Partnership for Food Safety Education at www.fightbac.org.

An Ounce of Prevention…

Go wash your hands. Any soap will do, along with warm water and 20 seconds of thorough scrubbing. Then, if you're ready to fix a meal, make sure everything that will come in contact with your food, such as utensils, countertops, and cutting boards, are as clean as your hands.

A few more bacteria-fighting prep tips:

- Wash everything in your kitchen with which raw

Flapping in the Breeze

Thorough hand washing doesn't always get rid of the germs. Studies show that still-wet hands can transfer up to 68,000 microorganisms. So before you touch anything, dry your hands for 10 seconds on a clean cloth towel or paper towel, then wave them in the air to dry for another 20 seconds. This procedure can cut the number of microorganisms by 99 percent.

meat juices come in contact: faucet handles, dish drainers, drawer handles.

- Don't return cooked meat to a container that previously held it raw unless it's been thoroughly washed with soap and hot water. That goes for utensils, platters, and other outdoor grilling implements you use, too.

- Don't pour marinades in which raw meat was soaked over cooked meat. If you intend to use marinade over your meat when it's finished cooking, set some aside before you soak raw meat in it.

Postcooking bacteria-fighting precautions are just as important as precooking preparation. Where bacteria are concerned:

- Warm water is their aphrodisiac. They'll multiply as fast as they can when you soak your dishes

for hours. If you're a soaker, make sure you change the water and clean the sink with a disinfectant before you do the washing.

- They love to congregate in dishcloths and towels. Use your washrags and towels only once, then run them through the wash on the hot cycle. Throw sponges in the dishwasher or wash them with hot water and soap after each use, since they won't survive the washing machine. You can also microwave your dishcloths and sponges for 60 seconds to kill *Salmonella* and *Staph*.

Pitch your sponge, though, when a good clean-

Vegetarians Beware

Don't think you're safe from that hamburger-loving *E. coli*, because you're not. Vegetables grown in soil fertilized by animal manure can be contaminated, too. Wash those fruits and veggies carefully.

ing doesn't get rid of the foul smell or it just plain looks disgusting. And, if you don't want the hassle of washing or replacing rags, towels, and sponges, switch to paper towels. It's expensive and environmentally unfriendly, but bacterially safe.

It Ain't Over 'Til the Thermometer Sings

You can't judge a book by its cover, nor can you judge whether a hamburger's cooked sufficiently by its color. At least 25 percent of all burgers turn brown before they're done, and when you bite into a juicy, brown, half-cooked burger, you could be swallowing a mouthful of *E. coli* (*Escherichia coli O157:H7*), a nasty little visitor that loves to camp out in ground meats. It causes bloody diarrhea, kidney failure, and, in extreme cases, death, all of which are high prices to pay for gobbling down some undercooked meat. You're not going to get rid of all the germs when you cook your food, but that's okay because most of them won't harm you. You stand the best chance of getting rid of the ones that can come back to haunt you an hour or two after you've eaten, though, by thoroughly cooking that burger, or any other meat or meat product you prepare. To do that, you'll need a standard meat thermometer. Ground meat needs to register 160°F, while ground chicken and turkey should be a little bit hotter, at 165°. Fresh beef, veal, and lamb need to be 160° for medium and 170° for well-done. Cook poultry breasts to 170° and poultry thighs, legs, and wings to 180° before you eat them.

Leftover Rules

You gotta love them. They're just sitting there, waiting for someone to eat

Picnic Perishables Can Poison You

That wicker picnic basket may look nice, but it's not intended for perishable foods. Without the benefit of cooling, its tag-along picnic guests can cause food poisoning. Carry picnic perishables in a cooler with ice, and keep the lid on it as much as possible. Stash it in the shade, too.

them. But they do come with their own precautions, because a little bad handling can turn those glorious leftovers into a gut-lurching nightmare.

The first absolute rule is that no perishable food can be left unrefrigerated for more than two hours—or one hour where the room or outdoor temperature exceeds 90°F. If you discover you've left the potato salad out too long, pitch it, or the bacteria that have started to feast in it may pitch something right back to you.

When you stash hot leftovers in the refrigerator or freezer, cool them quickly so the microorganisms don't have time to put on their party hats. Divide large portions into smaller portions and use shallow freezing containers to accelerate the cooling process. And cut leftover meat off the bones before refrigerating because they retain heat longer than the meat and become a bacterial breeding ground.

The second absolute rule is don't refrigerate leftovers indefinitely. You need to notice them before they turn green and take on a life of their own.

Egg-cellent Advice

For only a few pennies, an egg will provide 6 grams of protein and a boatload of important vitamins, minerals, and amino acids necessary to support life and growth. Unfortunately, they also have the dubious distinction of carrying *Salmonella enteritidis,* an intrepid little intruder that can cause fever, stomach cramps, diarrhea, and, in rare cases, death. The threat comes only when eggs are eaten raw, so don't eat raw eggs. Don't drink those "healthy" beverages made with raw eggs, either. And stay away from other foods traditionally made with raw eggs, such as Caesar salad dressing, hollandaise sauce, and homemade versions of mayonnaise, ice cream, eggnog, and cookie dough.

The good news is that pasteurized egg products can be substituted in many cases.

Here are a few more egg safety tips:

- Buy only refrigerated eggs. Make sure the eggs are clean and uncracked.

- Keep hard-cooked eggs, including Easter eggs, in the refrigerator.

- Don't freeze eggs in the shell. To freeze whole eggs, beat whites and yolks together. Egg whites can also be frozen by themselves. Use frozen eggs within one year.

Where the Bacteria Hide

Cutting-boards are one of the worst bacterial havens in the kitchen. Toss out any cutting board with cracks, crevices, or deep knife scars, because these are areas where the bacteria frolic. Disinfect the ones you keep with a capful of bleach added to a quart of water, and wash them with hot soapy water after each use. Ideally, use one cutting-board for meat products and one for produce, and don't interchange them.

- Don't leave cooked eggs out of the refrigerator more than two hours.

For more information, call the U.S. Department of Agriculture's Meat and Poultry Hotline at 1-800-535-4555 for a list of recorded topics.

Antibacterial Soap Overkill

Antibacterial soap does what it claims to do: kill bacteria. But government studies indicate that ordinary soap will do the job just as well. In fact, frequent use of antibacterial soap is contributing to the development of the growing number of antibiotic-resistant organisms, which is of increasing concern to medical professionals. Almost all the major infectious diseases are gradually becoming resistant to the drugs used against them. So use antibacterial agents sparingly to preserve the desired effect for when you need it.

Here are simple ways to achieve the same effect as an antibacterial agent:

- Use regular soap and hot water for hand and dish washing. Soap gets rid of bacteria simply by washing them away.

- Make hand washing a habit. Hands are the most common way germs are transmitted.

Brown Baggin' It

Whether you go with the traditional bologna sandwich or you prefer something a little more exotic, such as peanut butter and kumquat jelly, you probably want to make sure that's all you're eating when lunchtime rolls around. Follow these lunch box tips for the safest lunch:

- An insulated lunch box is the best choice, but if you

prefer the ol' brown bag, double bag it to keep the cold inside a little longer.

- Include a cold source, such as a couple of freezer gel packs or frozen juice boxes. Pack perishables between the cold sources.

- Keep your lunch out of the sun and away from other heat sources.

- Pitch perishable leftovers. Your gel pack won't stay frozen all day and perishables will spoil.

- If you like hot foods, take them in an insulated bottle. Don't pack your food in a plastic container to heat later, unless you keep it cold with a gel pack until it's time to reheat and eat.

- Never leave perishable foods at room temperature for more than two hours.

What's in That Drinking Water?

The source of your drinking water contains nearly 60 contaminants regulated by the government, not to mention animal carcasses, old tires, and if you're lucky, a pirate's chest full of gold. There is no such thing as pure water, and the end product that you drink, no matter what its source, didn't start out even close to being clean. It could have been contaminated with lead, arsenic, *Giardia,* or *Legionella,* all of which can

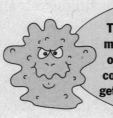

Beware the lurking bacteria. They're hiding in the cold spots in your microwaved food, and they could be a source of contamination. If your microwave doesn't cook evenly, rotate the food so everything gets its fair share of the rays. And stir, to mix all things evenly.

make you severely ill or even kill you if untreated. Some contaminants come from the erosion of natural rock, others from factory-discharged waste. Lead leaches in from old pipes, while pesticides find their way in from the soil. But municipal waters are doused with chemicals that clean them up for human consumption; rural well water can be treated as well.

What are those cleansing chemicals you drink every time you gulp down or cook with tap water? They're aluminum, chloride, copper, fluoride, iron, and manganese, to name a few. And do they hurt you? No, the amounts are regulated, and most have been assessed to have healthful benefits; fluoride helps prevent tooth decay, iron prevents anemia.

Because water standards differ from place to place, the only way to find out what's in your water is to call your water company and request a water-quality report. This will tell you what's on tap. Also, if you're concerned about water purity:

- Call your local water company or health department for the name of a reputable laboratory that can test your water. Don't rely on test results from someone selling water filters. They're usually "fixed" in order to make a sale.

- Check into filters. There are about 600 different brands on the market, so do your homework before you decide which is the best for you.

- Switch to bottled water. Unfortunately, it's not always what it's cracked up to be. For a list of water bottlers that meet international quality standards, visit the International Bottled Water Association Web site at www.bottledwater.org.

Risking It in Public

In the time it takes you to read this paragraph, someone was involved in an accident in a public place. An accident occurs every five seconds, and 20,000 people die each year as a result. But there's more at risk in public places than having an accident. When you're out and about, you're exposed to illnesses, chemicals, and many other dangers. Grim events for just sticking your big toe over your property line, aren't they? But going out in public isn't all doom and gloom if you know what precautions to take.

Waiter, There's a Bacterium in My Soup

Is your favorite restaurant a breeding ground for shigella or hepatitis A? Both come from poor personal hygiene—a trip to the bathroom without a good hand washing afterward. Think of *that* in terms of the food that's being cooked or served for you.

Shigella causes diarrhea and flulike symptoms, and it's estimated that a half-million cases a year are from some sort of fecal-oral contact. Hepatitis A, which is diagnosed about 200,000 times each year, causes liver damage. It gets to you via the same route as shigella—

Bacteria Shower

Disinfect your showerhead every week or so. It's a breeding ground for Legionnaires' disease. Use a teaspoon of chlorine bleach in a quart of water.

sometimes served right up on your dinner plate. Both are contracted in public places, including restaurants, and since many of us are eating nearly 30 percent of our meals in those restaurants, it's a good idea to ask yourself these questions (and run for the door if the answer is no):

- Are the waiter's hands and fingernails clean? Are they covered with cuts or burns? (If you can see the people preparing your food, ask the same questions.)

- Is this restaurant clean (menus, floor, plates, silverware, glasses)?

- Are there any signs of insects?

You have standards for cleanliness when it comes to preparing and serving your food at home, and you should never lower them when you eat out. Protect yourself by taking a good hard look around.

Hazards at the Pump

You probably know that gasoline is highly flammable, but did you know that it's not the liquid itself that burns? It's gasoline's vapor that ignites. Mix the right amount of oxygen, a spark, and a bit of vapor, and you've got a violent explosion. In fact, there's enough explosive power in one cup of gasoline to equal five sticks of dynamite.

Gasoline is still flammable even after it's dried on your clothes or skin. So be sure to change clothes if you spill gas on yourself, and wash your hands or any area of skin that has come into contact with the liquid.

But flammability isn't the only reason to wash your hands after fueling up. Gasoline contains benzene, a cancer-causing chemical. If you spill any on yourself while pumping gas, wash it off immediately with hot water and soap so the benzene doesn't absorb into your skin.

And while you're at the pump, stay there. If you climb back into your car, especially when the weather's cold and dry, scraping your feet across the floor carpet could cause a buildup of static electricity on your shoes. When you drag that static buildup back out to the pump, the sparking can ignite gas vapors that stay low to the ground, and boom, you've got a flash fire. If you get back into the car while it's filling, be sure to discharge the static electricity when you get out, before you touch the gas hose nozzle, by touching your car's outside metal, well away from the filling point.

Raunchy Restrooms

When you flush the toilet in a public restroom, the swirling water creates a fine mist that sends out

Pick a Stall, Any Stall

Some public bathroom stalls are cleaner than others. One study of men's bathrooms showed that people tend to use the middle stalls or the ones at the end, so your safest bet may be the first stall in a multi-stall bathroom. And if you have a choice, pick a bathroom that has two to four stalls. Bathrooms with only one stall or five or more stalls get heavy use and are more likely to be dirty.

disease-causing *E. coli* bacteria and other bugs that can cause diarrhea. So flush, then get away from the spray.

Many people have phobias about public toilet seats, but the real germ playground is the sink and faucet. You know where the hands were that turned that faucet on before you, and you can easily become contaminated if you don't take proper precautions. So turn on the faucet, wash for at least 20 seconds with soap and hot water, and use a paper towel to turn it off. Dry your hands on paper towels, too, because those hot air dryers and cloth towels on rollers are loaded with the things you're trying to wash off your hands. Then use the paper towel to open the restroom door so you can escape germ-free.

Keep Your Distance

Don't get too close to those beautiful July 4th fireworks in the city park. Stay at least a quarter of a mile away for safety's sake, as well as getting the best view. And if any part of an unexploded firework falls to the ground near you, don't touch it. It can still explode and cost you a couple of fingers. Call the fire department instead.

Sick-Building Blues

If your doctor hasn't been able to find the cause of your headaches; eye, throat, and nose irritation; dry cough; dizziness; nausea; fatigue; and difficulty concentrating at work, your office may be to blame. Yes, your building can make you sick, but it's not because you're just plain tired of being in it. Sick Building Syndrome (SBS) describes a range of acute health problems that seem to be linked to time spent in a building or in a particular part of a building. Chemical contaminants such as formaldehyde fumes from particle board products, biological contaminants like mold, and inadequate ventilation can all be contributing factors.

Solution: Leave the building for several minutes to shake off mild symptoms. Then discuss the problem with your employer. Better ventilation or thorough cleaning is often the simplest solution. So is switching to another office if the problem is limited to a particular area. In an extreme case, another job in a different building might be the cure.

Camping Safety

Do you know enough to brave the great outdoors for a day or two and survive? Here are four things you may not know.

1. The most common camp injuries are blisters, cuts, sprains, bruises, and fractures, not snakebites. Carry a first-aid kit and know basic first-aid procedures. If a snake does bite you, though, don't make an incision to suck out the poison. A little open sore in your mouth is a doorway for the poison to enter your system. Carry a snakebite kit and use the venom extractor.

2. During a lightning storm, the best place to seek protection is a dense forest located in a depression. But don't huddle under an isolated tree or a tree that's taller than adjacent trees; they attract lightning. If you can't find low ground, face away from the oncoming storm and squat down with your feet close together. This lessens your risk of sustaining injury from ground currents if lightning strikes nearby.

3. No unpurified water is completely safe, not even water from a crystal clear mountain stream. Take along water purification pills or a water filter (you can find them at camping

stores), and follow the instructions.

4. Any little creature wandering through the woods can have rabies, and every year more than 7,000 rabid animals are identified in the wild. If you are bitten, wash the wound with soap and water, then seek immediate medical treatment.

For more camping information, grab a copy of the *Boy Scout Handbook* or visit the Web site at www. scouting.org.

Man's Best Friend...

Can quickly become man's worst enemy when you greet and startle him in a public place. In fact, dogs are responsible for 4.7 million bites a year, of which 800,000 need medical attention. More than half of those bitten are children, 20 of whom die from the bites.

You and your children can avoid getting bitten. First, you have to realize that no matter how friendly and loveable your Fido is, the common everyday Fido you encounter on the street probably doesn't have the same temperament. Never approach a dog you don't know.

If that dog approaches you, however, don't run away screaming. It'll probably run after you. Instead, stand still and wait for it to walk away. If the dog knocks you over, roll into a ball and lie still. Whatever you do, don't look the dog in the eye. That's a challenge to fight, and you don't want to fight.

Don't bother a dog that's sleeping, eating, or caring for puppies. That's another invitation to fight. And, if the dog seems friendly and acts like it wants to be petted, let it sniff you before you make a move toward it.

Best advice: Just stay away. It may be cute, but it may also be vicious, and unless you know the dog, it's impossible to anticipate its reaction.

Caring for a Dog Bite

Your puppy has all its vaccinations, so if you get nipped in a playful romp it's not a big deal. But if a strange dog bites you, wash the wound immediately with warm water and soap, and apply a sterile dressing if the bleeding is excessive. Seek medical advice regardless of the severity of the bite if you do not know the status of the dog's vaccinations. For more information on dog bites, visit the Humane Society of the United States' dog bite education Web site at www.nodogbites.org.

Dial-a-Flu

Public phones connect you with more than the person you're calling. They can give you the bacteria and viruses deposited by a previous caller who touched, sneezed, or coughed on them. The solutions aren't very good if you need to use a public phone. You can carry a disinfectant with you everywhere you go and clean up the phone before you handle it, or you can avoid public phones altogether by carrying your own cell phone.

Book Germs

Library books can be germ carriers, too. You never know who has sneezed on them or what was on the hands that last touched them. After you read, wash your hands. A little of that antibacterial hand cleanser might be in order for long hours spent in library research.

On a Bicycle Built for One

Bicycling sure is popular today, whether for recreation, sport, or transportation—57 million Americans have taken up the call to pedal. Unfortunately, 900 of them are killed every year; 600,000 suffer serious injuries. Head injuries cause 75 percent of all the fatalities, but the good news is that a helmet will reduce the odds of head injury by 88 percent and facial injury by 65 percent. So wear that helmet!

Helmets may not be fashionable—or all that comfortable—but it's estimated that 500 bicycle fatalities and 150,000 injuries could be prevented if every rider donned a helmet approved by the Consumer Product Safety Commission. Here's how to do it the right way:

- Make sure the helmet's snug, but not too snug. If you can get a couple fingers between your head and the helmet, that's okay. If you can stick your fist in there, try another helmet.

- Sit the helmet on top of your head in a level position. It shouldn't rock back and forth or from side to side.

- Buckle the straps, and keep them buckled.

Lifesaving Helmets

Only 25 percent of children ages 5 to 14 wear a helmet when riding. But 97 percent of all children who are killed in bicycle-related accidents were not wearing helmets.

The Wheels on the Bus Go 'Round and 'Round

Every school day, 25 million kids board a school bus, and while school buses are the safest way to get

Move Back

The safest place to sit on *any* bus is in the backseat. Why? Most bus crashes are head-on collisions.

children to school, 33 kids die each year from school-bus-related injuries. The youngest riders, kids aged five to seven, are the most frequent victims. They are struck and killed outside the bus by a passing motorist or the school bus itself, usually in the "danger zone"—the area along the passenger sides and at the back of the bus. So, teach your children to stay at least 10 feet away from the bus and never to go behind it. If they drop something near the bus, tell them to ask the bus driver to help them pick it up.

Airing Your Dirty Laundry in Public

You take your clothes to the laundromat to clean them, but you can unwittingly pick up some nasty germs in the process. Dirty clothes, particularly under-garments, contain lots of harmful bacteria, including *E. coli*. An average load of wash can leave 100 million *E. coli* bacteria in the washing machine. The washing machine just spreads those bacteria around unless you use bleach and lots of hot water. Many of the bugs, such as *Salmonella*, hepatitis A, and rotavirus, survive the dryer.

Because people use the laundromat countertops to sort dirty and clean clothes, bacteria lurks there and can be transferred to your clothes when you fold them. And since wet laundry contains bacteria, you can get them all over your hands when you transfer clothes from the washing machine to the dryer.

Here's how to minimize your risk of infection:

• Don't touch your nose or mouth after handling wet

laundry. Wash your hands or use an antibacterial gel.

- Sort and fold your laundry at home or carry a bleach-based cleaner and use it on the laundromat counters before putting your clothes on them.

- Use bleach and hot water whenever possible to disinfect your clothes.

Wanderlust

Unfortunately, 5,000 pedestrians who love to go a-wandering are killed in traffic-related accidents every year, and 80,000 are injured. Most are children under the age of 16, older people, or people who were intoxicated. In fact, among adults who are involved in pedestrian accidents, alcohol is the major reason for death. One-third of pedestrians killed during the day are drunk. That percentage increases to one-half at night. Since you already know you shouldn't drink and drive, it's time to find out that you shouldn't drink and walk, either. Call a cab or friend instead of staggering along the street—or into it.

Beauty Beware!

Bad hair might not be your worst problem when you go to the beauty shop. If you have heart or circulatory problems, you could be at risk for a stroke when you slide your neck backward into the beauty parlor sink. The reason: Your neck arteries are squeezed, limiting blood flow to your brain. Most people won't suffer symptoms, but if you feel lightheaded as the beautician's giving you a scrub, or your face, neck, and arms get tingly, sit up immediately.

If you have a condition that might put you at risk, don't sit with your head stretched back into the sink for more than a few minutes at a time. Same thing goes

If You Survived the Beauty Parlor...

You may be facing another risk when you step out onto the street and breathe in the smog. If you have a heart condition, it's your heart, not your lungs, that may be most at risk from breathing the smog. When you suck in those tiny smog particles, they can change your heart rhythm, or even stop your heart from beating altogether. Studies have shown that when smog is at a *smog alert* level, more people die from, or are hospitalized for, heart problems. So if the smog level is high, stay inside or wear a mask.

for your dentist's office. Give those arteries a break, and sit up every few minutes.

How to Judge a Child Care Center

Two-thirds of all child care centers have at least one hazard that jeopardizes your child's life. And every year, 31,000 kids four years old and younger are treated in emergency rooms for injuries they received in a child care center. Seven die each year, too. So check this list before you drop off your child, and make sure you can answer "yes" to each question:

1. Is the crib in good condition, and does it exhibit a certification safety seal, have slats less than 2⅜ inches apart, and have a mattress that's firm and flat and fits snugly against the slats?

2. Have pillows, soft bedding, and comforters been removed from cribs in which babies sleep?

3. Does the day care provider know to put babies to sleep on their backs, not their bellies, to reduce the risk of Sudden Infant Death Syndrome?

4. Are safety gates in place to keep kids out of dangerous areas?

5. Are window blind and curtain cords secured by a tension or tie-down device that holds the cord tight in order to prevent strangulation?

6. Is the day care center equipped with smoke alarms, carbon monoxide detectors, fire extinguishers, electrical outlet caps, and antiscald devices?

7. Are cleaning supplies locked up? Medicines? Does the toilet seat have a lock on it, too?

8. Are the heaviest toys on the bottom shelves to prevent injury in case they fall?

9. Will the toy boxes open from the inside?

10. If the facility was painted prior to 1978, has all lead paint been removed?

11. Is the playground equipment safe?

Investigate. Ask questions. It's worth the extra time and effort it takes when it comes to the health and safety of your child.

Fountain of Death

That decorative fountain in the mall could be deadly if you breathe in any of the mist it sprays out. And the whirlpool spa on display at the home decorating center could be just as deadly if it's filled with water and bubbling out a fine mist. Why? They can be contaminated with *Legionella,* the bacterium responsible for Legionnaires' disease (LD). It loves to live and breed in water sources, especially those where water can stagnate, such as hot water tanks, cooling towers, and evaporative condensers in commercial air-conditioners.

It's estimated that 8,000 to 18,000 people come down with LD every year, and 5 to 30 percent of them die. Although we tend to think that LD occurs only as an outbreak, because that's when we hear about it, LD is most frequently a single, isolated case. Symptoms include fever, chills, cough, achy muscles, headache, and lethargy. Sluggish kidneys and pneumonia are also symptoms as the disease progresses. The good news is that the cure for LD is a simple antibiotic.

Hospitals Can Make You Sick

Every year two million people get zapped by bugs while they're patients in the hospital! These nosocomial (originating in the hospital) infections cause anywhere from 44,000 to 98,000 deaths per year. Patients in intensive care units are at the highest risk, especially for respiratory, urinary tract, and bloodstream infections. Catheters, intravenous lines, and ventilators are often the guilty parties that introduce the bug to the body. Patients with a surgical incision have the next highest risk.

Best defense: If you have to be hospitalized, make the stay as brief as possible. The longer they've got you, the more you're at risk.

On the Road Again

Booze isn't the only way to get in trouble behind the wheel. Sleepiness caused by common over-the-counter medicines and sleep deprivation are responsible for tens of thousands of car accidents every year.

In visual-motor reaction tests, people with sleep disorders score as bad, if not worse, than those who are drunk. Every year, 56,000 auto accidents result from sleeping or sleepy drivers; 40,000 cause non-fatal injuries, and 1,500 result in death.

Common over-the-counter antihistamines can cause more driving impairment than being drunk, too. Tests conducted on people taking diphenhydramine, an antihistamine that can make people groggy and put them to sleep, showed that during a standard driving test, they did worse than those who were classified as legally intoxicated. Diphenhydramine is found in common hay fever and allergy products, so read the labels before you buy.

Playin' Around

True or False? The playground was constructed for your kids, so you can assume it's safe.

The answer is False, and the 280,000 kids who are treated in emergency rooms for playground injuries every year are the proof that play equipment isn't always child-friendly.

Most injuries happen when kids fall off swings, monkey bars, climbers, and slides onto a hard, unforgiving play surface. Instead of nice, soft, loose-fill ground coverings such as sand, pea gravel, or wood chips, many playground floors are made of packed dirt or asphalt, neither of which will cushion a fall and prevent an injury. Grass doesn't provide sufficient cushioning either.

Kids love their playgrounds, but 20 die there every year. It's up to you, Mom and Dad, to make sure you recognize the hazards and guard your child against them.

Home-Unsafe-Home

It may be home sweet home, but that doesn't mean it's safe. In fact, the place in which you spend more than half of each day could be dangerous or even deadly. Each year, 7.3 million accidents happen in homes around the country. But accidents are only part of at-home risks. Your home is filled with toxic substances, allergens, and fumes—and you're probably not aware of many of them. And the security of your castle can be breached by unwelcome intruders as well. Luckily, home safety is mostly a matter of taking common-sense precautions.

Hidden Dangers in Common Household Products

Most of the time, product manufacturers don't tell you about potentially lethal ingredients, even if you study their warning labels with a high-powered magnifying glass. So here are a few ingredients you might find in your household products and problems they can cause, problems not listed on the label:

• Bug killers sometimes contain propoxur, which can cause nausea, vomiting, diarrhea, weakness, imbalance, blurred vision, breathing difficulties, increased blood pressure, and death. Buy either a brand without propoxur or a natural or herbal insecticide.

(Warning: Propoxur is also used in many flea collars. It could kill Fido or Fluffy if they're sensitive to it, as many pets are. The emissions from a flea collar are so close to a pet's face that they're inhaled directly into the lungs. Find a collar with natural ingredients or skip the flea collar altogether.)

- Mothballs are usually made with naphthalene or dichlorobenzidine, both of which can cause cancer or respiratory difficulties. Use cedar chips or blocks instead.

- Laundry detergents may contain 1,4 dioxane, a possible carcinogen. Switch brands if yours contains it.

- Cat litter containing crystalline silica is an eye and lung irritant. Try a natural brand made from pulverized paper.

Dangerous Plant Alert

Small children put everything into their mouths, and houseplants are no exception. This can be a serious problem when the houseplant is poisonous. There are 85,000 plant poisonings reported to poison control centers every year, and the flora munchers are almost exclusively children, whose developing bodies can make the ill-effects of plant poisoning much worse. The good news is that most

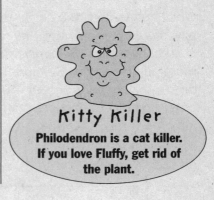

Kitty Killer
Philodendron is a cat killer. If you love Fluffy, get rid of the plant.

plants are not poisonous, and deaths rarely happen.

Azalea, bird-of-paradise, daffodil, holly, hyacinth bulbs, and mistletoe can cause heart, liver, and kidney damage, so be especially careful if you have those in the house. And Boston ivy, calla lily, Dieffenbachia, and philodendron can cause swelling of the mouth and breathing problems.

If junior did manage to snack at the houseplant salad bar, remove pieces of plant matter from his mouth immediately, then call your nearest poison control center. Never induce vomiting unless first instructed to do so by a poison control specialist. Some poisons cause even more damage as they come back up.

You're Not Going Crazy

If you suffer from a whole string of unexplained symptoms, such as headache, lethargy, depression, sleep problems, anxiety, difficulty concentrating, heat intolerance, and dizziness, and your doctor can't get to the

Don't Blame It on the Egg

Which came first, the chicken egg or the *Salmonella*? Actually, it was probably the *Salmonella*, since recent studies have shown that *Salmonella* from dirt sources is often more common than *Salmonella* from eggs. It turns up in dirt from your yard, dirt in your vacuum bag, dirt on your pets, and dirt on insects, and it's commonly cultured growing on a refrigerator shelf. That's not to say that it isn't in your eggs, because it could be. But *Salmonella* isn't just an egg problem.

bottom of it, it doesn't mean you're going crazy. You may have Multiple Chemical Sensitivity Syndrome (MCSS), which means you are allergic to any number of chemical-containing products. The list of potential allergens in your home includes aerosol air fresheners and deodorants, after-shave lotion, cologne, dry-cleaning fluid, floor and furniture cleaners, hair spray, bug spray, laundry detergent, marking pens, nail-polish remover, oil-based paint, and shampoo.

Because most doctors aren't diagnosing this yet, be your own detective and find out what's causing your symptoms.

- Keep a journal. Include symptoms and when and where they happened.

- Compare symptom outbreaks. Is there a similarity or something to connect them?

- Get rid of anything that seems to be the cause.

Switch to natural products wherever you can.

Formaldehyde in Your House

Formaldehyde is in your home, even if you don't have a science lab in your basement. It's used as a preservative or adhesive in many household products, including two that you probably own. If you have a home entertainment center that looks like wood but isn't, it's made from particle board, which is loaded with formaldehyde. So are the permanent-press clothes on your back. Formaldehyde is also found in some insulation materials and coated paper products.

Formaldehyde is used in such small amounts that it probably won't cause you any problems. It's emitted as a gas, though, and if you suffer from chemical sensitivities or have a specific formaldehyde intolerance, your symptoms will be burning eyes, nose, and throat; nausea; persistent cough; chronic headaches; chest tightness; and wheezing. Formaldehyde has also been identified as a possible carcinogen, but the verdict is still out on that one.

To decrease formaldehyde exposure in your life

- Buy "low-emitting" pressed-wood products; some are made with phenol formaldehyde.

- Use solid wood, not synthetic substitutes.

- Don't use foamed-in-place insulation or insulation marked "urea formaldehyde." Both emit the highest levels of formaldehyde gas.

- Wash permanent press clothes before you wear them. This gets rid of most of the formaldehyde.

Persian, Oriental, or Wall-to-Wall

No one's going to roll you up in it and drag you away, but your carpet could still be dangerous, especially if you suffer from asthma or allergies.

Mold Beneath Your Feet

Padding underneath carpeting is a breeding ground for mold and mildew because they are trapped with no place to go, even if the carpet on top is well-cleaned. Mold and mildew in carpet padding can cause serious allergies and trigger asthma attacks. To eliminate the possibility, there are two choices: You can buy a carpet with a pet-proof backing, which keeps soil right up on the surface, ready to be cleaned. Nothing will soak through to the pad. Or you can opt for a direct glue-down and skip the pad altogether. No pad, no place for anything to hide.

Humidifiers Can Make You Sick

Humidifier fever, a flulike illness, has been traced to microorganisms that grow in humidifier reservoirs, air conditioners, and aquaria. Symptoms include fever, headache, chills, muscle pain, and a general unwell feeling but don't include pneumonia, a symptom of Legionnaires' disease. Rigorous daily and end-of-season cleaning regimens, coupled with disinfection, are the only effective methods to eliminate the problem, according to the Environmental Protection Agency.

Whether they're made from natural or synthetic fibers, all carpets emit volatile organic compounds (VOCs), especially when the carpet is new. VOCs come from the glues used to hold the fibers together, not from the carpet fibers themselves. Carpets don't contain formaldehyde, however, which is the good news.

If you are very sensitive to fumes and odors, skip the carpet and stick to bare floors. Otherwise, to install a carpet with the least amount of pollutants:

- Buy carpet, padding, and adhesives with the green label of the Carpet and Rug Institute Indoor Air Quality Testing Program. They meet government standards for emissions of VOCs.

- Let carpet air for a day or two before it's installed.

- Ventilate the room in which the carpet is installed for 72 hours, when most emissions will have cleared out. Don't let babies or small children crawl on it until then.

Hold Your Breath!

Know what else you're breathing at home? Deadly chemicals, that's what. Here are four of the most lethal chemicals and what you can do about them.

CARBON MONOXIDE (CO)

CO is a colorless, odorless gas that prevents the delivery of oxygen to the body. CO results when fuels containing carbon are burned, including coal, wood, charcoal, natural gas, and fuel oils. CO poisoning is often misdiagnosed as flu or food-poisoning because it has some of the same symptoms: fatigue, headache, weakness, confusion, nausea, and dizziness. But flu or food-poisoning usually disappears quickly, while CO poisoning lingers. Untreated, CO poisoning can result in death; 1,000 people die from it every year.

To prevent CO poisoning

- Buy a CO detector. They're cheap.

- Do not use ovens and gas ranges to heat your home.

- Never leave a car or gas-powered lawn mower running in a shed, garage, or any enclosed space.

- Have your heating system, chimney, and flue inspected and cleaned every year, and make sure the flue is open if you use your fireplace.

- Inspect exhaust systems on your stove and heaters to make sure they're not leaking.

LEAD

You may be breathing a little lead dust without knowing it. It comes from deteriorating lead paint or the curtains and blinds that hang around it. It also comes from outside dirt that is dragged inside. Lead dust can land on woodwork, eating and playing surfaces, your child's clothes, and just about anything else inside your house.

In children, lead exposure will cause brain damage, kidney damage, and deafness and also affect growth because lead is absorbed easily into growing tissues. Lead will absorb into adult tissues, too, causing many of the same illnesses.

If your house was built before 1978, it could contain lead paint. Have it tested. Houses built after that won't have lead paint, but other lead sources, such as dirt, can still cause contamination. To be safe, dust suspected lead-painted areas daily and keep anything with which junior comes into contact especially clean, including toys. For more information, call the National Lead Information Center at 1-800-LEAD-FYI.

RADON

This is the second leading cause of lung cancer in the United States. Radon is found in dirt, and it's caused by the breakdown of uranium in rocks and soil. Nearly 1 in 15 homes have elevated radon levels, and it gets the credit for 14,000 deaths each year. There are no outward symptoms associated with radon; it just sneaks up on you. Testing for radon is easy and inexpensive, though, so go to the hardware store and grab a kit. For more information, call 1-800-SOS-RADON.

Fogger Beware!

The residue from pesticide foggers can remain in the room for up to two weeks even though the label says it's safe to enter the room within three or four hours. Don't fog a room where toddlers and young children live or play because the pesticide residue will cling to plastic toys and stuffed animals. It will cling to pet toys, too.

ASBESTOS

This is a mineral fiber that was used in insulation before 1970. If it is in good shape and not breaking apart, it's not a health risk. But when the asbestos begins to deteriorate and the fibers break apart, they are released into the air, putting you at risk for lung cancer, cancer of the chest and abdominal linings, and irreversible lung scarring.

Check your yellow pages for a professional in asbestos inspection and removal, but be very careful who you pick. Asbestos removal scams abound, and many who claim to be qualified are not. Check licenses and references.

More Indoor Pollution

Chemicals aren't the only indoor pollutants, and since you spend about 65 percent of your time breathing home air, some of those pollutants are going to get you, sooner or

A Growing Problem

Water-soaked carpet will begin to grow health-threatening mold and mildew within 24 hours. Clean and dry carpet thoroughly before that happens or consider having it removed and replaced. It can cause serious respiratory problems if you don't.

later. Most don't have to be harmful if you know how to control them.

DUST MITES

These microscopic critters feast on your dead, sloughed-off skin particles—even as you're reading this book. They congregate in areas where you spend a lot of time, such as your bed or your favorite recliner. To control them, control your environment. Avoid furniture that collects dust. Put your bedding in allergen-impermeable covers, and wash sheets and blankets at least once a week. Get rid of wall-to-wall carpeting and replace it with area rugs that can be washed. Since dust mites live in surface dust, get rid of dust-catchers such as knickknacks.

PETS

You love your furry pets, but something about them doesn't love you back. Contrary to popular thinking, it's their dander, not their hair, that causes allergies. If you have a pup, bathe it weekly and keep it out of your bedroom.

INDOOR MOLD

Mold grows in damp, humid areas and triggers allergies and lung problems. To prevent it, keep your bathroom, kitchen, and basement clean and dry. A dehumidifier can be helpful. Disinfect showers and other damp areas regularly.

Cosmetic Casualties

Some nineteenth century cosmetics contained lead and often killed the women who wanted nothing more than to look beautiful. Today, cosmetics are safer to wear, but they do come with their own brand of problems—usually allergic reactions. Beyond that, though, there are other cosmetic health concerns.

THE MOLDY OLDY

You've had that tube of lipstick for a couple years and it still does the trick. But it's been picking up all sorts of microscopic bad guys over time, so either use it up faster or buy a new one every few months.

STORE-TESTER CONTAMINATION

There's no telling where that store tester has been and what germs have taken up residence. Although cosmetics contain preservatives that destroy much of the contamination, it takes a while for them to kick into action after they've been used. At home they have hours or even a whole day to do their job. In a department store, there may be only a few minutes between uses, and that's not enough time to kill contaminants. So skip the tester and ask for a new sample.

For safer beauty

- Stash your cosmetics in a dark place. Sunlight destroys the preservatives that fight bacteria in makeup.

- Pitch the eye-makeup you used when you first came down with the infection or you could recontaminate, starting that infection all over again.

- Never resuscitate your dried-up makeup with a drop of water. Water causes the bacteria to jump up and multiply with all due haste.

Ten Things No Home Should Be Without

Do you have these items in your home? If you don't, be sure to get them!

1. Smoke alarms outside the kitchen (smoke and steam can set them off) and outside the bedrooms. Check batteries monthly, and replace alarms that are more than ten years old.

2. A fire extinguisher labeled ABC. Not every extinguisher will take care of every fire, but an ABC will.

3. Escape ladders installed for each room above the first floor. Buy them at a home center.

4. Emergency evacuation plan. Each room must have two escape routes—one through a door and one through a window. Hold a family fire drill twice a year.

5. Carbon monoxide detectors.

6. A radon testing kit.

7. Labels on shut-off valves for gas, oil, water, and electricity. Know where these valves are located.

8. A well-stocked first-aid kit. The Boy Scouts of America are the ultimate in preparedness, and here's what they suggest for your

Don't Move It

If a grease fire starts in a pan, don't move it. Moving the pan increases the oxygen flow to it, and this, in turn, can cause an explosion or flare-up. Instead, put on your oven mitt and carefully slide a lid over the pan. Then turn off the heat, and allow the fire to die on its own.

own kit: soap, roll bandages, adhesive tape, sterile pads, triangular bandage, gauze pads, adhesive strips, oral thermometer, scissors, tweezers, sunscreen, lip salve, poison ivy lotion, small flashlight with extra batteries, absorbent cotton, safety pins, needles, and ice packs. Also suggested: latex gloves, eye protection, antiseptic, and a resuscitation mask.

9. Disaster supplies as recommended by the American Red Cross: food and water for three days per person (one gallon of water per day per person), first-aid kit, clothing, bedding, tools (screwdriver, hammer, wrench, and other basics), flashlight, radio, extra batteries, medications, sanitation needs, and pet supplies (including water).

10. Emergency phone numbers posted by every phone.

Think Like a Burglar

It will take him less than 60 seconds to break into your house, and if you'll be so kind as to leave that spare key on the window ledge or under a rock, you'll cut his time in half. Your burglar thanks you for this because he's got another six million burglaries, minus one, to pull off within the next year.

One out of every ten homes is burglarized every year. To keep yours from being one of them, look around and see how easy it would be for *you* to breech your home's security. If you can do it with no sweat, think how easy it will be for a professional.

Check these out:

- Locks. Many burglars will spend no more than 60 seconds attempting to enter a home. If you leave your doors and windows unlocked, that's all it will take for him to slip right in. Burglars in almost half of all completed burglaries gained entry through unlocked windows and doors. Find the best locks for every door and window and use them.

- Flimsy doors. If one good kick will break it down, guess who'll be spending the evening in *your* house?

- Outside invitations. No lights or lights burning 24 hours a day, lots of shrubs, and a pile of newspapers. Guess what? You're an easy mark. Your house either has the perfect outdoor environment to hide a burglar or it's announcing that nobody's home. You might as well plant a

If You Meet Your Burglar Face to Face

Burglars do more than steal. They can rape, assault, and kill if they're surprised by someone coming home. Follow these tips to save your life:

- Don't go in if something looks wrong, such as a slit screen, open door, or broken window.

- If you're at home when someone tries to break in, get out, but don't put yourself at risk doing it. If you can't escape, lock yourself in a room with a phone and call the police. If you find yourself in the same room as the burglar, pretend you're asleep.

- Never confront your intruder. He could be armed.

flashing neon sign in the yard that says, "Hey guys! I'm burglar-friendly."

Decrease your chances of getting hit even more by installing an alarm system, getting a barking dog, and joining or starting a neighborhood watch program. Then go back and try to be your own burglar. Remember, if you can still get in, so can he.

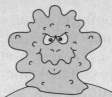

The More, The Riskier

The larger the household, the greater the burglary risk. Homes with six or more members have three times the rate of property crime of homes with one member.

Beware of Grandma!

You and your kids love her. She has candy and cookies and lots of hugs. But Grandma also has some things that can kill your kid.

Grandma's pills are a big threat to your children. They look like candy to toddlers, and they can show up anyplace in Grandma's house—on her nightstand, sitting on the edge of the bathroom or kitchen sink, or next to her favorite recliner. Almost 2.5 million children under age six are poisoned each year, and Grandma's medications account for about 500,000 of them. So check all her favorite pill places before turning junior loose in her house. And when she comes to visit you, stash her purse and luggage on a top shelf, out of junior's reach. Either, or both, could be veritable traveling pharmacies.

Poison, Poison Everywhere

More than 6,000 people die as a result of some sort

of poisoning at home each year, and 300,000 sustain disabling illnesses. And it's not only children who are poisoned. They are in the highest risk category, but adults between the ages of 25 and 44 are also at high risk because they fail to read and follow directions on medications and household chemicals. Follow this room-by-room safety checklist to prevent poisoning hazards in your home:

Doggy Dreck

Fido loves them, and they keep him from exercising his teeth on your furniture, but those pig ears, rawhide bones, and other "leathery" animal products he loves to chew can be infested with *Salmonella*. If Fido drags it out and buries it in the dirt, watch out for *E. coli,* too. Consult your vet for better choices in dog chews and toys.

BATHROOM

- Install childproof locks on cabinets storing medications, cosmetics, and cleaning products.

- Don't let junior see you take your pills, and never refer to them as candy.

- Read the instructions on the label before you take your pills.

BEDROOM

- Pitch the mothballs and have a cedar lining installed in your closet.

- Don't keep hair spray, cologne, nail polish remover, and other cosmetics where junior can reach them.

LIVING ROOM

- Hang coats out of junior's reach. You never know what's in the pockets.

KITCHEN

- Lock cabinets that hold cleaning supplies.

In Case of a Burn

Don't use butter, no matter what your mother told you. It seals in the heat and causes the burning to continue under the skin long after the surface burning has stopped. Instead, apply cold water. For a serious burn—one that causes swelling or blisters, chars, singes, or turns the skin leathery—apply dry-wrap gauze and seek medical attention. And never use ice to cool a burn. It can cause further damage to your skin.

- Never store food and cleaning products in the same cabinet.
- Keep everything in its original container.

Fire, Fire, Burning Bright

More than 135,000 fires are started in the kitchen every year, resulting in 40,000 injuries. Carelessness is usually the cause. People walk away from the stove or leave oven mitts or wooden spoons near a burner, where they can easily catch fire. Food in microwaves can catch fire, too. If you see smoke or flames coming from your microwave, unplug it and leave the door shut to smother the fire. If a fire starts in your regular oven, turn off the heat and keep the door closed.

The Big, Bad Outdoors

The sun's shining, the grass is growing, the birds are chirping, and you can't wait to get out and enjoy it all. But hold on! The sun can burn your skin to a crisp, the birds are singing because there are so many blood-sucking, poison-spewing insects to eat, and the grass needs mowing with what can be a dangerous tool. When you think about all the outdoor hazards, it can make you poke your nose right back inside and lock the doors. But with a little bit of information, you can do more than look out the window. Here's how to be safe in the big, bad outdoors.

Grill Smarts

Do you know what's lurking out in your yard? Danger! And it's not because your next-door neighbor is pitching a wild horseshoe. The following tips will help you enjoy a safer summer when you grill, whether it's in your yard, at the beach, or at the park:

• When lighting an outdoor grill, use an electric starter or barbecue starter fluid. Never use gasoline, kerosene, or other flammables; 5,400 people die as a result of outdoor grill accidents every year.

- Don't refresh your fire with more fuel. The fire could travel up the liquid's stream and burn you. Instead, fan your fire or add dry kindling.

- Wash hands or remove clothes that come in contact with starter fluid. A spark can ignite the fuel-soaked area.

Don't Get Zapped

To zap-proof your outdoor electrical sockets, make sure they're protected by ground-fault circuit interrupters. They cut off the current in case of an electrical imbalance or surge. Make sure your outside outlets are waterproof, too, and that any extension cords you plug into them are rated for outdoor use. It would be sad to plug Santa in next Christmas, when the snow is three feet deep, only to have him take an electrical hit and fry to a crisp.

Beat by the Heat

If the heat really gets you, you could die. When it's really hot, your body works double time to keep you cool, letting heat escape through sweat and exhalation of warm air. If your heat-escape mechanisms quit, first the blood flow to your brain will slow down and you'll feel faint. That's called heat syncope. Then your muscles will begin to ache, you'll feel nauseated and feverish, your skin will turn clammy, and your pulse will race. These are signs that you're in the second stage of a

Hot Stuff

Starter fluid can ignite under extremely hot conditions when left outdoors. Store it in a cool, locked cabinet.

heat attack, called heat exhaustion. When you become confused and lethargic and hyperventilate, you are suffering from heat stroke. You may also convulse or become unconscious. Heat stroke can be fatal. Your temperature may spike to more than 106 degrees, which is rarely survivable, but if you do survive, you've probably fried your brain and most of your vital organs.

Avoiding this mess is easy, though. Wear loose-fitting, lightweight, light-colored clothes when you're in the heat. Drink lots of water or sports beverages—more than you need to satisfy your thirst. Avoid caffeine, it's a diuretic. And don't drink alcohol, either. It, too, is a diuretic. And limit vigorous activities.

Texas Look Out!

All you Longhorns down there are at a greater risk of getting melanoma (skin cancer) than those North Star lake-lovers up in Minnesota because you have more sunlight than they do. More sun means more of those ultraviolet (UV) rays, and they cause premature aging, as well as other skin damage. But it's not just the sun that's putting people at risk for the most rapidly increasing form of cancer in the United States. It's exposure to any UVs, including those from tanning beds. To avoid those cancer-causing rays

• Stay out of the midday sun from 10 A.M. to 3 P.M.

• Remember this rule: Protect yourself from the sun when your shadow is shorter than you are.

• Cover up if you're out during the danger hours. Wear long sleeves and hats with a brim to protect your face.

• Apply one ounce of sunscreen to *all* exposed skin 15 to 30 minutes before you go outside. UV rays

When the Bell Rings

Alarms aren't just for school fires and home burglaries. There are all kinds of alarms to warn you of impending disaster. Here's a sampling of what's available. Try them— they could save a life.

- Door alarms let you know when your child is leaving the house.

- Gate alarms sound when the gate is opened.

- Infrared detectors sound when the area around the pool's perimeter is entered.

- Pool alarms placed directly on the water sound when something or someone enters the water.

- Child alarms are worn by kids; they sound when the child exceeds a certain distance from the parent base or when the alarm is submerged.

come in two types: UVA and UVB, both of which can cause skin damage and cancer. Some sunscreen products, primarily those with the lower SPF (sun protectant factor) numbers, only protect you from UVB, so choose a broad-spectrum product with an SPF of 15 or higher. Sunscreens with an SPF of 30 or higher provide the best protection.

- Select sunglasses that block at least 99 percent of both UVA and UVB rays. Wraparounds are the best choice to keep the rays out of your eyes. The next best choices are shades that fit closely. Three times more UVs will hit your eyes if they're loose than if they're close-fitting.

Are You at Risk?

Nearly 50,000 cases of malignant melanoma are diagnosed each year, and 20 percent of those diagnosed will die from it. The risk factors are

- Fair to light skin

- Family or personal history of skin cancer

- Lots of freckles

- Lots of outdoor time

- Sunburning easily

- Atypical moles or a large number of moles

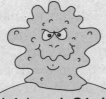

Kids at Risk

Studies show that when children have one or more blistering sunburns during their early years, their risk for developing melanoma increases dramatically.

If you have any of these characteristics, play it safe in the sun. For more information on skin cancer, visit the National Cancer Institute Web site at www.nci.nih.gov

How to Save Your Life

Checking your skin regularly for changes in moles can help you detect skin cancer before it becomes a killer. The best time to check is after a shower or bath, and the best place is in a well-lit room with a mirror.

First, make a mental map of all your moles. Don't be shy—you're not the only person with a mole in that embarrassing spot, so take a good look at it. Evaluate every mole for size, shape, texture, and color. If you're inclined to forget, keep a written record. Recheck every few months if you're not in a high-risk category; monthly if you are. Note any changes, and that means *any* change, because a changing mole can be a sign of cancer. See your doctor immediately. Skin cancers are highly treatable in their early stages, but if you wait, they'll spread, some even to your internal organs.

Self-Tanner Warning

If you choose to acquire your tan without the sun or trips to the tanning salon, that's fine. Self-tanning products are safe to use. But don't be misled; most don't protect your skin from ultraviolet rays. Check the label, and if you don't see an SPF number, you're not safe in the sun.

The Deadly Buzz

Mosquitoes are more than a nuisance; their bites kill millions of people each year. Most of those are in underdeveloped countries, where mosquito control isn't a government opera-

Insect Put-Offs

Mosquitoes and other insects are attracted to your body heat, exhaled carbon dioxide, perfume, and Hawaiian prints. You can't do much about body heat and exhaled carbon dioxide, but avoid perfumes and other sweet-smelling potions, and stick to plain, light-colored clothes when you're in mosquito territory.

tion. But, some of those "foreign" mosquito-borne diseases, such as malaria, do slip into the United States occasionally. So if you notice unusual symptoms after a bite, such as fever, fatigue, headache, stomach pain, and muscle aches, call your doctor. Malaria is highly curable with early treatment.

Encephalitis, an inflammation of the brain, is always a risk during mosquito season, which is summer. Symptoms include headache, muscle stiffness, fatigue, sore throat, and breathing difficulties. Because encephalitis is a virus, there is no cure. But don't despair. Early medical treatment can prevent serious complications and death.

To deter mosquitoes

• Burn citronella candles during outdoor activities, such as picnics.

• Wear insect repellent when outside for long periods of times. Those labeled "deep woods" offer better protection.

• If you live in a mosquito-infested area and don't want to sleep under mosquito netting, dab on a little camphor. Mosquitoes hate it.

• Mosquitoes live and breed near stagnant water, so if you have some on your property, clean it up and spray.

Bee Sting Strageties

Bees won't kill you unless you're allergic to their sting. They'll just leave you with a present—a stinger with a venom pouch embedded in your skin.

If you do provoke Mr. Bee, scrape the stinger away from your skin with a fingernail. Try not to squeeze the venom sac. Then wash the area with soap and water and apply a cold pack for 15 to 20 minutes.

If you're one of the two million Americans who are allergic to bee stings, you may require allergy shots, and you'll probably need to carry doctor-prescribed medication that will counteract the allergic reaction. If you've never been allergic before, it doesn't mean you never will be. Insect bite allergies can start at any age, and when they pop up, it's usually within minutes.

Knowing what happens when a bad bug bites can

save your life, so if you're bitten and develop any of these symptoms shortly after, get to a doctor:

- Nausea
- Dizziness
- Stomach cramps and diarrhea
- Itching all over your body
- Hives
- Wheezing and difficulty breathing

The Eight-Legged Guy

Most spiders are harmless and won't bite you, unless you've really made them mad. The two poisonous exceptions are the black widow, commonly found in warm regions, and the brown recluse, which lives in the Midwest and, to a lesser extent, in the East.

These three tips will help protect you from unfriendly arachnids:

1. Know your deadly spiders on sight. The female black widow has a black, shiny body and a distinctive red hourglass marking on her belly. The recluse, often called the fiddleback, bears the mark of a violin on his back.

2. Know what their poisons will do. If the black widow gets you, you'll feel

How to Remove a Tick

Despite what you've heard, burning a tick off or coating it with fingernail polish or petroleum jelly will not remove it. Instead, use tweezers or your fingers (only if they're protected by a tissue, paper towel, or rubber gloves) to pull it off. Grab that tick close to your skin and pull it straight out without twisting. Or, lift it up and pull it parallel to your skin. Don't pop the tick once it's out. What oozes out can still spread infection.

a dull, numbing pain at the bite site within 15 minutes. Soon after, you'll experience muscle stiffness, vomiting, sweating, and dizziness. Symptoms from the bite of a recluse, however, don't show up immediately. It can take as long as eight hours before the bite mark swells to a red blister that looks like a bull's-eye. Fever, weakness, vomiting, joint pain, and a rash follow.

3. Know what to do. Get to a hospital as fast as you can. If you don't, the bite could be fatal.

Tick, Tock...It's Not Your Clock

You've heard about Lyme disease. It's carried by the deer tick, found primarily in the Northeast, Midwest, Mid-Atlantic, and West Coast regions, and it affects nearly 14,000 people each year. Early symptoms include a rash at the site of the bite within seven to ten days. The rash expands out, leaving a clearing center. Fever, headache, muscle and joint aches, and swollen lymph glands are also common. Untreated symptoms may progress to sleep disorders, heart problems, and death. But Lyme disease is easily treated and highly curable with antibiotics.

Lyme disease isn't the only tick-borne disease in the forest, though. Ticks can also cause:

• Rocky Mountain Spotted Fever, found in the East, South, and West

• Babesiosis, found in the Northeast and West Coast areas

• Ehrlichiosis, found in the South Atlantic and South Central areas

• Tick-Borne Relapsing Fever, found in the West

• Colorado Tick Fever, found in the West

• Tularemia, found throughout the Southeast,

ZzzzzzzZap!

Splat!—That's what you have to worry about when the bug zapper zaps. Recent studies have shown that when some bugs fry, they explode and send innards, parts from other bugs they've eaten, bacteria, and viruses up to seven feet away. Either lay that zapper to rest or keep it away from your picnic table.

South Central, and Western regions

- Tick Paralysis, found in the West and East

Tick-borne illnesses are treated with antibiotics, but not every antibiotic will cure every tick disease. So no matter what you've heard, don't self-treat with leftover penicillin or whatever your doctor prescribed the last time you were sick because it might not cure what the tick gave you.

Barefoot in the Grass

About 400,000 people are treated in emergency rooms every year for injuries from lawn and garden equipment. Twenty-five thousand of them are injured on riding mowers, 75 of whom die. So when you're pushing a lawnmower, riding a garden tractor, or even just handling a rake, make sure you protect yourself.

The following are mowing safety tips:

- Always wear shoes.

- Wear long pants to protect your legs from flying debris.

- Wear eye protection. One million eye injuries happen at home each year, and 90 percent could have been prevented with eye protection.

- Remove sticks, rocks, and other debris before mowing. They can be thrown from under the mower deck at 200 mph if you run over them.

- Never pull a mower toward you—or you could chop off a few toes. Always be sure to push it away from you.

- Don't refuel while the engine is still hot. It could spark and ignite the gasoline.

Do You Really Need Pesticides?

Studies show that up to 80 percent of all lawn treatments are unnecessary, which is a lot when you consider that we dump 70 million pounds of pesticide on our lawns every year. There are natural and safer alternatives. But if you're a poison person, follow some basic rules to protect yourself or you'll end up being the one receiving treatment.

- Wear protective gear: gloves, mask, and eye protection.

- Spot treat. There's no need to go overboard by spreading poison everywhere.

- Don't apply pesticides when it's windy.

Watch Where You Step

Lawn pesticides can be tracked into the house for a week after they've been applied. So take off your shoes after you've been plodding through the green stuff, and don't let Fido romp in it for a week, either. Also, make sure junior doesn't have access to the lawn. Young children are particularly susceptible to pesticide poisoning. Ask guests to leave their footwear at the door or place a doormat at the entrance and ask them to please wipe their shoes on it.

- When you're through, wash yourself, plus everything you wear.

For more information about pesticide use and to find out which pesticides are on the government recall list, visit the Environmental Protection Agency's Office of Prevention, Pesticides, and Toxic Substances at www.epa.gov/pesticides.

Recognizing Jack Frost's Bite

Jack will go for your fingers, toes, heels, hands, nose, and feet in sub-freezing temperatures if you're not careful. The first signs of frostbite are red, numb, and slightly swollen skin. Blisters will follow as the frostbite worsens, and eventually your skin will become pale and hard. Frostbite starts with a dull ache that gets progressively worse. At the worst stage, though, pain may decrease and even disappear.

Bundle Your Fingers

Mittens are better than gloves, even if they're not as convenient to wear. They trap heat from your other fingers and don't limit your circulation.

Frostbite threatens your limbs. Advanced frostbite often results in amputation because the affected body part has simply died. If you're going to be in the cold for long periods of time, protect yourself.

- Eat plenty of food—it produces body heat.

- Drink liquids—they increase your blood volume, which means your extremities won't freeze quite so fast. Believe it or not, your body can actually demand more water in the winter if you spend prolonged periods in the cold.

- Don't rub frostbitten extremities—it causes

more tissue damage. Instead, submerge extremities in water that's not quite hot to the touch, about 104 to 108 degrees.

- Take an aspirin—it will prevent blood-clotting.

- Get medical help as fast as you can.

Shoveling Out

If you have coronary artery disease, are middle-aged or overweight, or are physically inactive, you need to follow some simple rules when shoveling snow.

Take the following precautions suggested by the American Heart Association:

- Layer your clothes to keep warm.

- Wear a hat or scarf on your head. Protect your hands and ears, too.

- Go at it slowly. Physical exertion and cold weather do mix, but together they can put an overload on your heart. So take your time, don't exhaust yourself, and take frequent breaks.

- Don't drink alcoholic beverages to fortify yourself before the big shovel. It draws heat away from the body's vital organs, which makes them susceptible to damage.

- Watch out for the warning signs of a heart attack: uncomfortable pressure in your chest; chest pain; pain spreading to your neck, shoulders, or arms; light-headedness; fainting; sweating; nausea; or shortness of breath.

The best life-saving advice: Consult your physician before picking up the shovel.

The Medical Maze

If you don't have a medical background, it's a tough trip through the medical maze. Nearly 100,000 hospitalized patients die every year as a result of a medical error. And drug errors are responsible for 7,000 deaths annually. With more than 10,000 brand-name drugs and 7,700 generics, it's essential to know whether you're getting the right medication. Here's how to take yourself out of the lineup for medical and drug errors—as well as some additional advice about protecting your health.

It's All Greek to Me

Actually, it's Latin that's used on your prescriptions. And while you don't have to be a Latin scholar, it helps to know what your doctor is writing so you can check what you're getting from the pharmacist. This little Latin lesson will help keep you out of the statistical column called "medication error."

Rx: prescription
ac: before meals
bid: twice a day
gt: drop
hs: at bedtime
od: right eye
os: left eye
pc: after meals
po: by mouth

prn: as needed

q3h/q4h: every 3 hours/ every 4 hours

qd: every day

qid: 4 times a day

tid: 3 times a day

If your prescription reads "tid," but the label on your medication says "four times a day," you know there's been a mistake.

Five Life-Saving Questions for Your Pharmacist

It will take a couple of minutes to ask these questions, but you might reduce that medication death count to 6,999 by doing so. Isn't that worth the extra effort?

1. What's the name of the medication and what's it supposed to do? Your doctor should have already told you the answer, so this is just your way of double-checking.

2. When and how do I take it? The answer to this question is also written right on the prescription, so compare it with what it says on your medication's label.

3. Can I take it with the other medications I'm already taking? Your pharmacist can do a quick computer analysis for the answer.

4. Should I avoid alcohol, other food, or certain activities? Make sure your druggist puts the warning labels right on the bottle.

5. What are the side effects?

Don't hesitate to ask your pharmacist questions. After

Weighing the Dose

Medication dosages are normally calculated for someone weighing 155 pounds. If you're significantly above or below that weight, you may be receiving too much or too little of the drug. Make sure your physician is prescribing the proper dose for your weight.

all, it's your life you're protecting.

Online Drugs: Convenient, but Safe?

There are hundreds, maybe thousands, of Web sites selling prescription drugs, and it's hard to tell which ones are legitimate. There are even a few selling products that are not approved for sale in the United States. Of course, that "pharmacy" may not even be in this country. And some online outlets are helping customers sidestep their physicians by requiring only the completion of a questionnaire, not a doctor's prescription, to purchase medications.

So what's an online customer to do?

• Check with the National Association of Boards of Pharmacy to see if an online dealer is licensed and in good standing at www.nabp.net.

Fastest Relief!

To receive the fastest relief from your nonprescription painkiller, buy the liquid variety. It gets into your system faster than the pills, which have to dissolve in the stomach before being absorbed into your body.

• Don't buy from online pharmacies that will sell a prescription drug without a prescription.

• Don't buy from a site that won't let you talk to a pharmacist.

I Have to Do What With Those Suppositories?

If you'd read the label, you'd have known they aren't just big, waxy pills you take with a huge glass of water. And you're not alone in your dangerous ways. Up to 50 percent of those who take prescription medicines don't read label instructions, either. But the directions are there for a very good reason—your health—and they shouldn't be taken lightly.

If the directions say to take the pills for ten days, eight days isn't good enough, even if you're feeling better. Ten full days are what you need to make sure that bug you have is beyond resurrection.

And timing is important to many medications. Some pills should be taken only in the morning, while others are for bedtime. Morning blood pressure medication taken at night, for instance, can cause eye damage, and your ulcer can kick up if you take your nightly ulcer pills in the morning. So get out those spectacles and take 30 seconds to read the label. You'll make your health problems much easier to care for, and you could even save your life.

Attack Your Heart Attack!

About 300,000 people die from heart attacks each year because they didn't get medical help quickly enough. Seventy-five percent of those who survive with little or no permanent damage received some form of anticlotting therapy within an hour of the onset of symptoms. (Heart attacks are a result of a clot blocking blood flow to certain

Buzz Saw Warning!
If you're a heavy snorer, it could indicate that you have sleep apnea. When people with sleep apnea come out of anesthesia, they may not breathe sufficiently, which can cause heart and brain damage. If you're a heavy snorer, tell your anesthesiologist.

areas of the heart.)

One of the best and most handy clot dissolvers, if you're experiencing the warning signs, is a regular-strength aspirin. Take it immediately, chewing it up so it will dissolve and start working faster.

Heed these heart attack warning signs:

- Uncomfortable pressure, fullness, squeezing, or pain in the center of your chest that lasts more than a few minutes.

- Pain spreading to the shoulders, neck, or arms.

- Chest discomfort accompanied by lightheadedness, fainting, sweating, nausea, or shortness of breath.

Know Your PSA

Every year, 185,000 men are diagnosed with prostate cancer, and 40,000 will die. With early detection, though, it's a highly treatable cancer. A simple blood test called Prostate Specific Antigen (PSA), drawn from a vein in your arm, can determine if you have, or are at risk for, prostate cancer.

Here's how to understand the numbers when your doctor gives them to you:

A healthy prostate produces prostate cells, and a reading of less than four is normal. The lower the number, though, the better. Levels between four and ten indicate the presence of prostate cancer, normally in a beginning stage and limited to the prostate. A reading above ten shows progression of the cancer, but it's still usually limited to the prostate until the PSA hits fifty, which means the cancer is now spreading throughout the body.

Normally, a prostate exam consists of your doctor's finger probing a very indelicate place, but ask about adding a PSA test to your yearly physical, just to be on the safe side. It saves lives, but many doctors aren't prescribing them yet.

This One's for You, Ladies

More than 180,000 women are newly diagnosed with breast cancer in the United States every year, and about 40,000 die from the disease annually. The mammogram is a simple X-ray procedure that can detect breast cancer early—and save your life. For the best mammogram

- Use a facility that specializes in or performs many mammograms each day.

- Ask to see a U.S. Food and Drug Administration certificate.

- Ask for your old mammogram films if you change facilities. Take the originals, not copies, because they have better film clarity.

- Avoid having your mammogram the week before your period, when your breasts are the most sensitive.

Plain English

A new law requires that all mammography facilities send you a written summary of the mammogram report. It must be written in easy-to-understand language, not all that medical mumbo-jumbo.

If you haven't heard the results from your doctor within ten days, call and ask. No news is not necessarily good news.

Got a Roll?

If you have a little roll around your waist, get rid of it. The roll, plus a significant weight gain around age 30, puts you at a higher risk of dying of breast cancer. Any weight gain of more than 11 pounds counts. And it also puts you at higher risk for many other diseases, such as endometrial cancer, gallbladder disease, hypertension, diabetes, and arthritis.

But don't despair. You can change your risk factors by altering your diet and exercising.

Women who already have breast cancer can benefit from reducing the roll, too. Losing some of it increases their odds of survival.

More Than a Contraceptive

Birth control pills taken for six years or longer lower the risk of hereditary ovarian cancer by 60 percent. Even women who have taken them for three years or less decrease their odds by 20 percent. There's a comparable benefit against non-hereditary ovarian cancer, and the pill may even reduce the risk of uterine cancer and pelvic inflammatory disease.

Skip the pills if you smoke or have high blood pressure. Heart problems or stroke could result.

Attack of the Killer Clot

When a clot goes to the brain and shuts off the blood supply, the result is called a brain attack, or stroke. Every minute in the United States, someone experiences a stroke. About 160,000 of the nearly 750,000 who do have strokes every year die as a result. Of the survivors, up to 18 percent will have another stroke within a year. That rate drops to 10 percent each year after that.

Everyone's heard the term "stroke," but almost 20 percent of all people over 50 can't name a single symptom. So, here are the top five:

1. Sudden numbness or weakness in the face, arm, or leg—usually limited to one side of the body.
2. Sudden confusion and trouble speaking and understanding. Mouth may droop on one side.

Get Thee to a Hospital

The old myth was that a stroke isn't treatable. But it is, and the quicker you get to the hospital, the better your odds of recovery. Fifty-eight percent of all stroke victims wait at least 24 hours to seek help; the median time from the onset of a stroke until medical help is sought is 13 hours. Not good! New treatments and medications are reducing the effects of stroke and even reversing the condition altogether, but they must be administered within 90 minutes to do any good. So don't wait, not even an extra minute or two. The time it takes you to debate the pros and cons of seeking medical help could mean the difference between permanent disability and a return to normal life.

3. Trouble seeing in one or both eyes.

4. Difficulty walking, loss of balance, dizziness.

5. Sudden stabbing headache.

Belly Up to the Cow, Boys

Milk may cut your risk of having a stroke. In fact, some studies indicate that men who drink milk regularly reduce their risk of stroke by half. There's no conclusive reason for this,

but it may be that men who drink milk are more likely to have a healthier lifestyle. Even so, perhaps wearing that little white mustache is worth a try.

A Little Calcium for the Ladies, Too

Calcium kicks premenstrual syndrome (PMS) right in its symptoms. Twelve-hundred milligrams (mg) of calcium a day may have a significant effect on bad moods, bloating, food craving, and pain. And since most women don't consume enough calcium, there are additional benefits to making sure you get the 1,200 mg. Calcium strengthens bones and lowers blood pressure.

The best way to get your calcium is by eating calcium-rich foods, such as low fat dairy products, dark green leafy vegetables, and calcium-fortified foods. Add a supplement if you need to, and always keep your daily intake below 2,500 mg. If you have a personal or family history of kidney stones, check with your doctor before taking calcium supplements.

Is It Safe to Help?

The Good Samaritan Law, which is in effect in many states, protects a passerby from being sued later on when he stops to give medical assistance. The only exception is when care or treatment given goes beyond rational first-aid guidelines. To find out if your state has this law, call your local medical association.

Phone Gossip Can Be Deadly

The way you hold your phone can cause a mini-stroke. Cradling it between your head and shoulder, especially if you're into marathon conversations, can compress a blood vessel in your skull and cut off circulation.

To prevent a stroke, switch the handset from ear to ear often, use your hands to hold the receiver, switch to a headset, use a speaker phone, or send e-mail.

If you use a digital cell phone, you're probably not going to have long conversations because of the cost. But you do have to worry if you have a pacemaker. Digital cell phones can temporarily turn a pacemaker off or cause it to speed up your heart rate. So if you have a pacemaker, use an analog phone. And regardless of the cell phone you use, don't keep it in a pocket over your heart when it's turned on. Those cell waves and your pacemaker waves don't get along when they're close together.

Remember This Word– Autologous

One person in 2,500 picks up a blood-borne illness through a transfusion, even though blood supplies are safer now and new screening techniques are filtering out most of the bad stuff. That's because tests are not completely foolproof; contaminated blood does slip through once in a while. And there's also the possibility that you could get the wrong match in the hospital. With the exception of the universal donor blood type O, blood type must be exactly matched. Reactions to unmatched blood can be anemia, shock, and death.

To protect yourself against blood-borne illness, make an autologous donation. That means you donate your blood to yourself. The most common autologous donation is done prior to surgery. You go to the blood bank, a technician draws and stores your blood, and then it is sent to the hospital when you're ready for it. Some blood banks will, for a fee, freeze and store your blood for several years. Another method, called cell salvage, traps blood that leaks out during surgery and recycles it back into your body.

If surgery is in your future, ask your surgeon about an autologous donation.

The Seven Signs You Should Never Ignore

Each one of these symptoms could indicate a serious problem—or even that

When Being a Universal Donor Doesn't Pay Off

Your type O blood is all the rage when someone needs a donation, so you go to the head of the line. But if you need an organ transplant, the line stops before you even get to it. Your universal type O organs can be used for anyone who needs a transplant, but you can use only another type O organ. Here are some surprising statistics:

- Type O patients wait 4–5 months longer than others for a liver.

- For heart transplants, type O patients wait 2–4 times longer.

- The chance of dying while waiting for an organ to become available is 22 percent with type B, 35 percent with type A, and 50 percent with type O.

death is imminent. Call for help immediately if you're experiencing any of these or if you see them in someone else:

- Difficulty breathing

- Chest or upper abdominal pain

- Fainting or sudden dizziness

- Coughing up or vomiting blood

- Sudden severe pain anywhere

- Bleeding that won't stop

- Severe or persistent vomiting

Saving Yourself

Choking happens. You're alone and that jumbo hot dog gets stuck in your windpipe. You cough and it won't come out, then panic sets in. To make sure you're not counted among the 2,800 people who die as a result of choking every year, here's how to give yourself the Heimlich Maneuver:

- First make a fist, then place it thumb-side against your stomach, just above your navel.

- With your other hand, grab hold of your fist and press it in and upward with quick, sharp thrusts until the hot dog is dislodged. You can also press your abdomen, just below your ribs, against the back of a chair, table, sink, or railing and thrust against it until the food is dispelled and you're breathing again.

The Universal Signal

You're in the restaurant and the man seated at the table next to you is clutching his neck between his thumb and index finger.

This is either an indication that he didn't like the veal parmigiana or that he's choking on it. Before you attempt anything, ask him, "Are you choking?" If he can answer or cough, that means air's getting into his lungs and you don't have to do anything. If he can't, proceed with the Heimlich Maneuver.

For an adult:

1. Stand behind the person and wrap your arms around their waist.

2. Make a fist, then grasp it with your other hand and place your thumb just slightly above their navel.

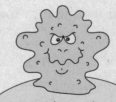

No Slapping!

Never slap a choking victim on the back. This can move the lodged food and cause it to wedge in the windipe even tighter.

The Heimlich for Drowning

The initial reaction when saving someone from drowning is to administer CPR, but that isn't the proper first response. Remember this: Before you do anything else, get the water out of the lungs. Use the Heimlich Maneuver. The death rate of drowning victims who were first administered CPR went from 40 percent to 3 percent when the Heimlich became the first response to drowning endorsed by the American Red Cross.

3. Thrust your fist into their abdomen in an inward and upward motion.

4. Thrust five times, then check the victim and adjust your position if necessary. Repeat until the food is dislodged.

For an infant:

1. Lay the baby face up on a firm surface or stand baby up on your lap facing away from you.

2. Place middle and index fingers of both your hands below baby's rib cage and above navel.

3. Press into baby's upper abdomen with a quick, upward thrust. Be careful not to squeeze the rib cage.

4. Repeat until the object is dislodged.

Pumping a Little Too Much Iron

Too much iron can kill you. We all need iron in our diets, and iron supplements are stocked on pharmacy shelves everywhere. But just because they're there doesn't mean you should take them. Too much iron in your system can lead to a condition called hemochromatosis, which occurs when your body can't get rid of the excess. It builds up in your organs, mainly your liver, and can destroy it. Too much iron can also lead to heart failure, diabetes, and cancer.

Before you decide that you need additional iron in your diet, consult your physician. A simple blood test will determine whether you do or don't.

Best Time for Surgery

No surgeon is likely to admit that some times are better than others for surgery. But the fact is that, unless you need emergency surgery, there are some days and times you should avoid altogether.

Worst times:

- Any afternoon after 3 P.M.: Your doctor is thinking about everything that needs to be done before going home.

- Friday afternoon: weekend's coming.

- The day before or after a holiday: party time or party recovery.

- June–July: The next generation just graduated from medical school and they're on the loose.

Best times:

- Morning, first on the schedule.

- Tuesdays, Wednesdays, and Thursdays: no weekend distractions.

More Scheduling Know-How

When your surgery is scheduled, ask if your physician is on the regular schedule for that time slot. If you find the doctor's on call (on standby for an emergency), your surgery could be bumped or delayed. If timing is important, avoid scheduling on an on-call day.

On-call days can be helpful, though, if your hip's killing you but your surgeon has a six-week waiting period before there's an opening in the schedule to replace it. Many times, a surgeon will not schedule regular surgeries for on-call days. Ask for a surgery slot on the next on-call day, but be prepared to wait if there's an emergency.

Prevent Mistakes Before They Happen

It may not be a pleasant comparison, but you should think about your doctor the way you think about your plumber. First you'd check out the plumber's credentials, then you'd ask him what's wrong and how he intends to fix it. And you'd certainly establish the price, method of repair, and the timetable before he started working. But do you do as much with your doctor?

These are important questions to ask your doctor:

1. Why do I need this procedure? Be sure you are convinced before you agree.

2. Is there an alternative? Often there is, and it's your right to know.

3. Will you be the one doing the procedure? You never know, since you're asleep. But many physicians employ "ghost" surgeons—usually experienced residents—to do their work.

4. Will you be there the entire time? Some cut and run to the next procedure, leaving you in the hands of someone else.

5. How many times have you done this procedure? You don't want to be the first.

6. When was the last time? You don't want that answer to be ten years ago.

7. What can I expect after surgery? Doctors are often noncommittal, but you need to know if you're destined for a rehab center, home, or six weeks recovery on a tropical beach.

8. What are your fees? They're often negotiable.

And here are some important questions to ask your hospital:

1. What's your nosocomial (originating in the

hospital) infection rate? If they won't tell, ask your board of health.

2. If you're having an outpatient procedure, ask how emergencies are handled. Most clinics and outpatient settings have standard emergency equipment, but check first to be safe.

3. How many times a year is this procedure done in your hospital?

No Chewing

Stomach contents and anesthesia don't mix, and the more you have in your stomach before surgery, the greater your risk of serious complications, including vomiting and aspirating that vomit into your lungs. That's why you're told not to eat or drink before surgery. But don't chew gum, either. Studies show that those who chew gum before surgery have 50 percent more stomach contents.

Ready, Set, Go!

When you're packing your bags for a trip, you need to include some common sense and caution along with your wardrobe. Otherwise, you could end up like Little Red Riding Hood, who naively assumed that the wolf wouldn't get her. But he's out there, waiting for the unsuspecting traveler. And he has plenty of opportunity, since 100 million U.S. households take 685 million trips each year, traveling 827 billion miles. Knowing how to beat the wolf before he pounces is the first step in a safe, healthy journey.

Leavin' the Country?

You could be stranded on foreign soil if you get sick. Many medical insurance policies don't cover travel abroad—and that includes Medicare. Check your policy before you go. And while you're at it, check the fine print for emergency transport back to the United States. If you need it, your policy might not allow it.

And, now that you've had all the exotic immunizations, don't forget about the basics, such as polio and tetanus. Don't show up at the dock only to have your boat sail away without you because you overlooked them. Check your vaccination status with your physician and call the Centers for Disease Control (CDC) Travelers' Hotline at 888-232-3228 or visit the Web site at www.cdc.gov to see what you need for the country to which you're traveling.

Warning!

It's not always safe to travel where you want to travel when you want to go. We're talking terrorist threats, bomb threats to airlines, bioterrorism, political uprisings, and more. For the most current information about a particular country's travel safety, including road and aviation situations and medical facilities, visit the U.S. State Department Web site at www.travel.state.gov/travel.

Cruising Cleanliness

Diarrhea and other gastrointestinal woes are not uncommon on cruise ships. The reasons: food-borne contamination associated with typical buffet serving lines, over-taxed sewage systems, and a lot of people in a relatively small area. All of these can spread billions of germs, causing tummy troubles you can't blame on seasickness. Some ships seem to produce more problems than others.

Logging in Without a Home Computer

Oh, no! So much good information available online and you without a computer. Try your local library. Most have computers available for public use at no charge. Or visit a university library. They have computers available, too. And if you don't know how to "log" onto the "Web," or what all that www dot stuff is about, ask a librarian.

The CDC's Vessel Sanitation Program conducts routine inspections of cruise ships, including their water supplies, spas and pools, food, personnel hygiene, and general cleanliness. If you're going on a cruise, check out your ship's sanitary rating at www.cdc.gov/nceh/vsp. A rating of 86 or better is acceptable. Less than that . . . well, you decide.

It Must Be Something I Ate

Sure it is, and it's called giardiasis, or more commonly, tourista, and it will demand you visit every bathroom you encounter on your vacation. Travelers get it from a change in drinking water, as well as overeating and the typical vacationer's "I'm on vacation and I'll eat when I feel like it" changeable dietary schedule. Part of the problem, though, is the food we consume—native dishes and things we'd never consider eating at home, like those crunchy cicadas that are so popular in Cambodia. But you're on vacation, so what the heck. The result is a queasy gut, a green-around-the-gills feeling, diarrhea, and time spent in the washroom instead of sight-seeing or relaxing on the beach. But it will pass—about 15 minutes before you catch the plane to go home!

A little caution, though, will help keep your gut from roiling.

• In areas where sanitation is bad, avoid salads, uncooked veggies, unpasteurized milk, and milk products.

• Eat only cooked food, and even then, only while it's still piping hot.

• Peel your own fruit.

• Avoid street food vendors.

• Drink bottled water or soda. Avoid coffee, tea, and other drinks originating with tap water unless the water has been boiled first. Skip the ice cubes, too. And check the bottle seal. A big scam in many tourist areas is to refill the bottle from tap water and sell it to another customer.

- Brush your teeth with bottled or boiled water.

From a bacterial standpoint, alcoholic beverages are safe to drink.

When You Shouldn't Fly

Don't even think about flying if

- you've had a heart attack within the past month. Cabin air has about 25 percent less oxygen than the air you breathe on the ground, which is damaging to a healing heart.

- you've had surgery within the past two weeks. Air pressure changes can split your incision wide open.

- you've been scuba diving within the past 24 hours. Reduced cabin pressure can cause the bends.

- you have a serious and chronic lung condition such as asthma. The decreased oxygen content of cabin air can be life-threatening.

- your hypertension (high blood pressure) is not controlled. Cabin-pressure changes can raise your blood pressure to stroke levels.

- you have severe anemia. Your body is already lacking oxygen since you

Aisle or Wing?

If you're pregnant, where you sit on the plane can make a huge difference in your comfort level. Aisle seats at the bulkhead offer the most space, but a seat over the wing will give the smoothest ride.

Too Young to Fly

Don't take junior on that plane until he's at least six weeks old. Until that time, the alveoli (air sacs) in his lungs don't work to capacity and he could suffer severe breathing problems. His ears are also extremely sensitive to cabin pressure changes, which can collapse his eustachian tubes.

don't have sufficient red blood cells to carry it. The decreased cabin oxygen can cause further oxygen deprivation.

- your epilepsy isn't well controlled. Constant pressure changes could trigger a seizure.

If you have these conditions and must fly, first consult with your physician.

The Safest Seat

Where you sit on an airplane can make a life-or-death difference. Don't plant yourself in the window seat next to the emergency exit. It could limit your escape options and endanger your life from people trampling over you trying to get out. Also, if the exit next to you jams, you could be trapped. The best seat is on the aisle, close to the over-wing emergency exits. You'll be near several other exits, which will give you better odds of escaping, and getting out of your seat will be much easier.

Don't fall victim to economy-class syndrome, either. The lack of leg room can cause circulatory problems, which can lead to the formation of potentially fatal blood clots in your legs. Remedy: Buy a first-class seat or ask to be moved to a wider seat. Get up and move around every half

Injuries in the Sky

Air turbulence is the leading cause of nonfatal, in-flight injuries, bumping and banging 60 people each year. You'll recognize them. They're the ones not wearing a seat belt, even though their flight attendant has informed them that for safety's sake seat belts should be worn at all times when seated.

hour, too, just to keep your blood circulating.

Tip: Ask for an aisle seat in which your prominent hand is on the aisle. You won't feel quite so confined since it's not wedged in next to someone, and you'll be able to relax more easily.

Junior's Life-Saving Carry-On

Your child's car seat could protect him from a turbulence injury or even save his life during a plane crash. The Federal Aviation Administration *strongly* suggests that you take a car seat on board with you and strap junior into it. Make sure it carries an aircraft

approval rating and that it's 16 inches wide so it will fit in most seats.

Children under the age of two aren't required to have their own seat, but many airlines offer deep discounts to encourage parents to buy one. That way, junior can be strapped into a child restraint system for a safer flight.

These are the rules for child restraint systems (CRS) on aircraft:

- Kids under 20 pounds go in a rear-facing CRS; those between 20 and 40 pounds in one that faces forward.

- Booster seats and harness vests are forbidden.

- CRS devices must be in window seats.

Head Cases

What's that behind you, resting its head against the airline pillow on which you're resting your head? The answer is anything that was on the previous flier's head or in his hair, including lice, seborrhea (crusty, yellowish-brownish-greyish dandruff), drool, and sneeze souvenirs. Airline pillowcase changes are infrequent—only a couple times a day if you're lucky, even though the plane you're riding on has made several flights. Carry your own pillowcase or travel pillow to avoid sharing the previous seat occupant's gunk.

Dry Air Miseries

Dry airplane cabin air can be deadly. It's dried out by anywhere from 80 to 98 percent, which means the air you're breathing contains only 2 to 20 percent of normal humidity. This desert-dry air doesn't usually cause problems beyond dry skin and thirst. For people with certain chronic health conditions such as heart disease and respiratory illnesses, however, dry air can lead to dehydration, which in turn can cause respiratory distress and heart palpitations. Here's how to keep dry air from causing problems:

- Drink a glass of water for each hour you fly.

- Stay away from diuretic beverages such as coffee, tea, cola, and alcohol. Instead, drink water and juices.

- Stretch your legs often and elevate them, if possible, to prevent blood clots. If dehydration becomes severe, blood can pool in your lower legs and become a real clot risk. This is especially important if you're pregnant.

Buzzzzz, Buzzzzz, Buzzzzz

Airplanes have other travelers besides the ones who pay for the ride, and some countries require that the nonpaying traveler be killed. That means the paying customer gets sprayed.

"Disinsection," the process of spraying the passenger compartment with insecticide while passengers are present, kills insects such as mosquitoes and fruit flies. While the sprays used internationally have been deemed safe by the World Health Organization, they may cause problems for some. Be aware that you'll probably be sprayed when you travel to Latin America, the Caribbean, Australia, and various South Pacific islands.

If you have questions about disinsection on your flight, or what disinsection agent will be used, contact your travel agent or the airline. Call your physician with health concerns if you have pesticide allergies.

How to Survive a Plane Crash

Most people, about two-thirds, do survive commercial plane crashes. The other third might have survived had they known what to do during a crash. So, if it looks like your plane is going down—and when a crash is imminent there usually *is* time to react—increase your survival odds by

- putting on your seat belt and adjusting it as tightly as you can.

- going over your mental list of exits and choosing your escape route.

- removing pens, pencils, dentures, belt buckles, eyeglasses, high heels, and anything else on your person that can cause injury.

- emptying your bladder to reduce the possibility of injury to internal organs.

- moistening something to tie around your mouth or nose, such as a shirt. Use any liquid except alcohol, including your urine, if you have to. *This is very important since most crash deaths are fire or smoke-related.*

- covering your head with a pillow. Then cross your arms over your calves and grab your ankles OR cross your wrists, with palms facing forward, and place them between your head and the seat in front of you. In this second position, slide your legs forward until they touch the seat in front of you or the luggage underneath.

After the crash, get out as fast as you can and

- don't wait to be told. Immediately unfasten your seat belt and get to the nearest exit.

- don't take any possessions.

- don't crawl, even if there is smoke. You'll get trampled. Keep your head down, though.

- when you find your exit, check outside the nearest window to make sure you won't be jumping out into a fire. If you see fire, go to the exit at the opposite side of the plane.

Nasty Hotel Habits

Your plane landed safely and it was a good flight, but now you're exhausted and all you want to do is get to

The Safest Floors

For fire safety, the best rooms are between the 4th and 6th floors (fire ladders can't reach above the 6th floor), nearest the emergency exit, on the front or most visible side of the building.

the hotel and climb into bed for a nap. Don't just crumple in a heap on top of that bed the minute you arrive, though. That bedspread wasn't cleaned after the last guest or even the one before that. And don't pull back the bedspread and flop down on the blanket. It wasn't cleaned, either.

In fact, sheets and pillowcases are the only parts of your bedding that get a regular washing. Everything else upon which you sleep rarely sees the laundry. All of it, according to several studies, has proved itself filthy, encrusted with everything from food and saliva to blood and semen. So has the carpet on which you walk barefoot.

The best remedy is to carry a can of disinfectant spray and give everything, including the phone, a good dousing. Think twice about using the coffeepot that's in the bathroom. If it's near the toilet, it's getting a bacterial shower

every time the toilet is flushed. If you do use it, wash it with soap and hot water first. Then think about those glasses and the ice bucket sitting on the back of the toilet.

Even the cleanest hotel room isn't clean. A better choice is to stay at a small private inn or bed and breakfast.

How to Survive a Hotel Fire

Surviving a hotel fire takes a little know-how. First, don't assume that the hotel sprinkler system will save you. It's estimated that up to 85 percent of U.S. hotels don't have them at all. So be prepared for the worst, and if it happens, use the following tips to get yourself to safety:

- Feel the door with the back of your hand before you step into the hall. If it's hot, stay in your room. If it's not, open it, drop to your knees, and crawl to the exit (*not the elevator*)—only if the hallway is clear of smoke. If it's not, slam the door shut.

- Stay on the same side of the hall as the exit. Head down the stairs, and if you encounter smoke, stop, turn around, and go back upstairs. Find a smoke-free corridor and cross the building to another exit.

- If you're trapped in your room, let someone know. Call the hotel operator or, better yet, dial 9-1-1. Hang a bedsheet out your window, too.

- Fill the bathtub with water. Wet towels and bedding and stuff them around doors and vents. If the walls are warm, bail water onto them with your ice bucket.

- Lean the mattress against the door and secure it there with the dresser. Keep it wet.

- Place a wet towel over your mouth and nose to help filter out smoke and heat.

- If you see fire outside your window, yank down the curtains to keep them from going up in flames.

Don't Let Your Neck Snap

Question: What happens when your body goes one way while your head and neck go the other, then snap back together?

Answer: You succumb to neck injuries, which occur in two-thirds of all auto accidents.

You can save your neck, though, if your head restraint is positioned correctly.

- When you drive, your head restraint should reach as close to the top of your head as possible and not less than 3.5 inches below the top of your head. The higher it is, the more protection it provides.

- Make sure it touches the back of your head but not your neck.

- Keep the back of your seat as close to vertical as possible.

Lighting the Way

Keep a flashlight next to your hotel bed. It can light the way through unfamiliar territory during an emergency.

Tall people, whose heads roll back over the top of the restraint in a crash, are most at risk for a neck injury.

Necessary Nuisances

Seat belts wrinkle your clothes and can be uncomfortable, which may explain why only 70 percent of us wear them, but they do save lives—more than 8,000 a year. So buckle up and follow these guidelines:

- The shoulder strap should cross the collarbone, and the lap belt should fit low and tight.

- Don't slip your shoulder strap behind your back or under your arm. This can be dangerous in a car with an airbag. Airbags come at you at 200 miles per hour, and the shoulder strap keeps you from flying forward into the force.

Airbags can kill, espe-cially small children and people who don't wear their seat belts properly. But they do save 1,000 lives a year. So put your kids in the back-seat, since it's the safest place for them. And follow these safety tips:

• When driving, sit at least ten inches away from the steering wheel. This is the deployment distance of an airbag. If you're short and sit closer to the wheel, try pushing your seat back and tilting the steering wheel forward. You can also raise the seat or sit on a cushion. Do whatever it takes, but maintain that ten inches.

• On the passenger side, push the front seat back as far as possible and sit no closer than 30 inches from the dashboard.

Convertibles and Cancer

You probably won't get sunburned in your car unless you hang an arm out or you're in a convertible. But low-level skin damage from the sun does happen, and it accumulates over the years, causing aging and life-threatening skin cancer. Since 1990, windshields have been partially treated to block the ultraviolet radiation that causes cancer, but side and rear windows are not. So protect your sun-exposed areas with sunscreen or long sleeves if you intend to travel for long hours during the day.

It's Simple, and It Can Save Your Life!

Keep something in your car that will break the window glass. Safety glass is impervious to a lot of bumps and hits, so don't count on kicking it out, even with those killer heels on your cowboy boots. The time it takes to get into position and land several good blows could be fatal if your car gets caught in a flash flood or other deep water. A tire iron, hammer, heavy-duty flashlight, or other heavy *metal* object will shatter glass in an emergency. Whatever you choose, keep it within easy reach—in the glove compartment or underneath the front seat.

Strappin' in the Kiddies

Never, ever, put kids in the front seat until they are tall enough for their feet to be flat on the car floor. Stick kids in the back and use a rear-facing infant seat until they reach 20 pounds, then switch to a forward-facing seat. When they hit 40 pounds and are four years old, switch them to a booster seat. Keep them there until they're at least six years old and can fit safely into the regular seat belt.

When mom and dad buckle up, their kids are buckled up 87 percent of the time. When mom and dad aren't buckled, junior and his siblings are buckled up only 24 percent of the time.

Your Traveling Emergency Kit

It may take up some trunk space, but a traveling emergency kit can save your life. The following basic supplies should be included in your kit:

- First-aid manual and kit
- Flashlight and extra batteries
- Spare clothes, shoes, blanket
- Bottled water, nonperishable snacks (replace or restock every few months)
- Pocket knife
- Radio with batteries
- Road flares
- Shovel
- Matches in a waterproof container (You can buy them where camping supplies are sold.)
- Emergency candles
- Booster cables
- Sand or kitty litter to provide traction

Also, consider keeping a cell phone in the car. It can be a real life-saver.

The Wrong Moves Can Be Deadly

If you're going to get stranded, it's most likely to happen in the winter. If you slide off the road or end up in a blizzard, don't panic. There are ways to manage the situation to keep yourself safe.

- Turn on your flashers.
- If visibility is poor, stay in your car.
- Run your engine intermittently to stay warm: on 15 minutes, off 15 minutes.
- Crack the window to guard against carbon monoxide poisoning.
- Grab those emergency supplies from the trunk when you need them.

How to Avoid Road Rage

It can happen to anyone, anywhere, anytime, and the result can range from an unfriendly gesture to death. Road rage is as old as Ben Hur's angst during his chariot races. But unlike Ben, who knew when the race was on, we don't know when road rage will come after us. Follow these tips to protect yourself against it:

- Avoid eye contact.

- Don't use the horn unless you absolutely have to, then do so sparingly.

- Get out of the way.

- If you're being followed, drive to a public place.

- Never pull directly abreast of the next guy at the stoplight.

- Don't gesture back, yell, or antagonize.

- Report road rage to the police immediately—on a cell phone during the incident if you can.